Digital Storytelling in Health and Social Policy

As digital life stories continue to assume more and more significance across a range of institutions, so too does their potential to bring into focus once marginalised and neglected voices. Breaking new ground by reframing multimedia life stories as a resource for education, public health, and policy, this book challenges policymakers, professionals, and researchers to reimagine how they find out about and respond to people's daily lives and experiences of health, disability, and well-being.

The book develops theoretical, methodological, and practical resources for listening to digital stories through a series of carefully selected international case studies, from dementia care education to campaigns in the UN to ban cluster munitions. The case studies explore and illuminate different ways that digital stories have – and have not – been listened to in the past. The authors expose the great potential as well as the complexity of using powerful personal stories in practice. Together, the case studies highlight that processes of listening to, learning from, and making use of digital stories involve unavoidable processes of reinterpretation, recontextualisation, and translation which have significant ethical and political implications for storytellers, listeners, and society. In mapping and theorising the movement of stories into new contexts of policy and practice, the book offers a critical lens on the widely celebrated democratising potential of digital storytelling and its capacity to amplify marginalised voices.

Digital Storytelling in Health and Social Policy develops an authoritative and original re-conceptualisation of digital life stories and their use for social justice ends, and will be important reading for researchers and practitioners from a range of backgrounds, including social policy, digital media, communication, education, disability, and public health.

Nicole Matthews lectures in media and cultural studies at Macquarie University in Sydney, Australia after having taught at universities in the United Kingdom (UK) for over a decade. In the early 2000s she began writing about the early uses of autobiographical video on broadcast TV, from *Video Nation* to *You've Been Framed!* Since then, she has been part of a number of collaborative research projects exploring the way that people use visual and electronic media to tell stories drawing on their own life experience. This work has included research on the way young Deaf people use video for storytelling and searching the web, and the evaluation of a UK project run by disability charity Scope which brought together stories written for very young children by disabled people and their families with illustrations and animations by art, multimedia, and design students. As well as her long-standing interest in auto/biographical media, Nicole has published on popular genres of print, broadcast, and electronic media and the politics and practice of higher education.

Naomi Sunderland lectures in the School of Human Services and Social Work and is an active member of the Queensland Conservatorium Research Centre and Menzies Health Institute Queensland at Griffith University, Brisbane, Australia. Naomi has an extensive background in participatory, creative, and community-based research in the areas of health, well-being, and arts-based community development. She has collaborated on many storytelling and health-related research projects including: the 1000 Voices Disability Life Stories project; a social determinants of health evaluation of the Scattered People asylum seekers and refugee music group; the Sensory-Ethnography of Logan-Beaudesert project; and a participatory intercultural evaluation of multi-arts work with Barkly Regional Arts in the Northern Territory. Naomi teaches in the First Australians and Social Justice team at Griffith University and specialises in topics around transformative intercultural and immersive education, equity, and diversity. Naomi has a PhD in applied ethics and human rights from the Queensland University of Technology. She has worked in government and non-government organisations and universities in Canada and Australia. She has published widely on the topics of health promotion partnerships, music and well-being, disability and happiness, and transformative ethics. Naomi is also an active singer, songwriter, and performer, and has released several albums of work internationally.

Routledge Advances in the Medical Humanities

New titles

Medicine, Health and the Arts
Approaches to the Medical Humanities
Edited by Victoria Bates, Alan Bleakley and Sam Goodman

Suffering Narratives of Older Adults
A Phenomenological Approach to Serious illness, Chronic Pain, Recovery
and Maternal Care
Mary Beth Morrissey

Medical Humanities and Medical Education
How the Medical Humanities Can Shape Better Doctors
Alan Bleakley

Learning Disability and Inclusion Phobia
Past, Present and Future
C. F. Goodey

Collaborative Arts-based Research for Social Justice
Victoria Foster

Person-centred Health Care
Balancing the Welfare of Clinicians and Patients
Stephen Buetow

Digital Storytelling in Health and Social Policy
Listening to Marginalised Voices
Nicole Matthews and Naomi Sunderland

Forthcoming titles

The Experience of Institutionalisation
Social Exclusion, Stigma and Loss of Identity
Jane Hubert

Bodies and Suffering
Emotions and Relations of Care
Ana Dragojlovic and Alex Broom

Digital Storytelling in Health and Social Policy

Listening to Marginalised Voices

Nicole Matthews and Naomi Sunderland

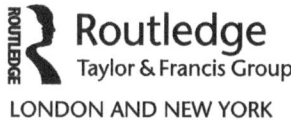

Routledge
Taylor & Francis Group

LONDON AND NEW YORK

First published 2017 by Routledge

2 Park Square, Milton Park, Abingdon, Oxfordshire OX14 4RN

52 Vanderbilt Avenue, New York, NY 10017

Routledge is an imprint of the Taylor & Francis Group, an informa business

First issued in paperback 2019

British Library Cataloguing in Publication Data
A catalogue record for this book is available from the British Library

Library of Congress Cataloging in Publication Data
Names: Matthews, Nicole, author. | Sunderland, Naomi, author.
Title: Digital storytelling in health and social policy / Nicole Matthews and Naomi Sunderland.
Description: Abingdon, Oxon ; New York, NY : Routledge, 2017. | Includes bibliographical references and index.
Identifiers: LCCN 2016048031 | ISBN 9781138024502 (hbk) | ISBN 9781315775708 (ebk)
Subjects: | MESH: Patient Participation | Narration | Public Policy | Health Promotion
Classification: LCC RA427 | NLM W 85 | DDC 362.1--dc23
LC record available at https://lccn.loc.gov/2016048031

ISBN: 978-1-138-02450-2 (hbk)
ISBN: 978-0-367-34917-2 (pbk)

Typeset in Times New Roman
by Taylor & Francis Books

For Rory, Surya, and Phil

Contents

Illustrations

Figures

Tables

Preface

It has been seven years since the two of us began talking about how listening to personal digital stories might prompt social change. We had both, in quite different ways, been involved in projects that sought to amplify the voices of people who experience marginalisation using narrative and digital media. As a new parent of a disabled son and an academic, Nicole had become involved in a UK National Lottery-funded project, run by the disability charity Scope, which aimed to get the publishing industry to include disabled characters in illustrated stories for young children. Disabled writers, and families of disabled children, developed fictional stories that were taken to art, design, and multimedia students to turn them into books, videos, and games. The political and interpersonal conflicts and silences that became evident in this project prompted much thought around the value and the difficulties of listening across difference.

After having the razing experience of growing up in a country town that was divided by racism, Naomi went on to study communication and applied ethics and human rights. She then worked in government and non-government settings and universities, as an advocate for social justice and public participation in policy processes. Naomi joined our colleague Professor Lesley Chenoweth in establishing the online 1000 Voices Disability Life Stories project at Griffith University in 2009, the first in a series of storytelling projects of which she was part. When we met at the Discourses and Cultural Practices conference held in Sydney, Australia in 2009, Naomi was presenting on the topic of the "missing discourses" of joy and happiness in disability policies and was contrasting this peculiar absence with the many expressions of joy, happiness, and flourishing that were present in people with disabilities' depictions of their own lives in and on their own terms. For us, this was an example of the many strengths of personal storytelling and the vital information it could reveal about people's lived experiences for policymakers and practitioners alike.

As we undertook research and publishing activities together, we began to develop our collective knowing in response to digital storytelling across geographical, disciplinary, and life experience boundaries. While Naomi was embedded primarily in a faculty of health and working within a school of human services and social work setting, Nicole was embedded in a department of media, music, communication, and cultural studies working primarily within the field of media studies. While one discipline favoured empirical research, practice frameworks, and practical outcomes, the other prioritised deep theorising, historicising, and philosophy. Over the years we have sought to both manage and mine the disciplinary divergences of our work to bring a kaleidoscope of perspectives, approaches, and thoughts to bear on digital storytelling and listening.

While we each bring diverse disciplinary resources to our shared table, we also share a deep commitment – alongside many of our colleagues – to using personal stories – digital and otherwise – to reshape unjust or under-informed representations and understandings of "others". This has included reshaping our own unjust or under-informed perceptions on many occasions. As we worked together on the 1000 Voices project between 2009 and 2014 in particular, we realised that sustainably reshaping unjust perceptions of others isn't so easy. This made us move more and more towards investigating the parallel processes of listening and responding to stories as a vital element in digital storytelling practice for social justice. We found that inviting people to tell stories about their experiences and sharing those stories publicly are perhaps not so difficult. Many of the people involved in the children's stories project Nicole had worked on in the UK and the 1000 Voices Disability Life Stories project viewed themselves as writers, as activists, and sometimes as both, and were passionate about telling stories to enable social change. In contrast, getting powerful people in industry, the professions, and government – and even students who might one day take up the roles of policymaker, professional, or business leader – to not just listen *but also actively respond* to personal stories seemed much more difficult. So, we thought, what is the good of asking people to tell their story if no one is listening?

This book aims to start a conversation about the complex and often challenging realities we and others have experienced when asking people to listen and respond to personal digital stories. To this end we have spoken with digital storytelling practitioners, advocates, policymakers, and academics from around the world during the preparation for this book. Our conversations have informed not only the case studies presented in this book, but also our evolving understandings of the complexities and realities of listening and responding to digital stories in health and social policy and practice settings. Our own contributions to the conversation via this book are of course partial and shaped by our own histories, stories, and positionality. We are both academics working in Australian universities. We are bound by the conventions of our practice in terms of the ways we wield and work with knowledge artefacts such as peer-reviewed journal articles, media sources, and personal stories. Yet, while we are speaking to an academic audience in terms of our professional accountabilities and heritage, our hope is that this book will be of direct use to health and human services practitioners, policymakers, digital storytellers, digital storytelling facilitators, and students as well as our academic colleagues. While this book's specific focus on listening – the way digital stories are shared, circulated, taught, attended to, and used – will often lead us to focus on certain things over others, we hope that this book will complement the important work that we all do in supporting people to create, share, and listen to stories.

Acknowledgements

We would like to acknowledge and thank the following colleagues and friends who have generously read and commented on this manuscript during its development including: Donna McDonald, Greg Hearn, Jane Simon, Steve Collins, Kate Rossmanith, Usha Harris, Marilyn Casley, Ruth Barcan, and Justine Lloyd as well as Nicole's wonderful dad Chris Matthews.

We would also like to thank our research partners and academic colleagues who have offered valuable feedback on case studies shared in this book including: Ashley Currie, Brad Currie, Allan Luke, Kathy Mills, John Davis-Warra, Annette Woods, and Elizabeth Kendall.

The book has been greatly enriched by the presentation of early drafts at seminar series and conferences. We are particularly grateful to Dimitri Eleftheriotis and Amy Holdsworth from the University of Glasgow; Cate Watson, Fiona Kelly, Richard Ward, Julie Christie, and Jane Robertson from the University of Stirling; Havi Carel from Bristol University; Mandy Rose and Gillian Swanson from the University of Western England; Lucy Burke from Manchester Metropolitan University; John Keady, Emma Ferguson-Coleman, and Sarah Campbell from Manchester University; Hamish Fyfe and Karen Lewis from the University of South Wales; Mark Dunford from the University of East London; Tanja Dreher from the University of Wollongong; Anna Poletti from the University of Utrecht; and Kylie Cardell and Kate Douglas from Flinders University for enabling immensely productive discussions around the themes of digital storytelling, learning, and health over the past decade. Exchanges with Kathryn Knight over the period of her candidature as a PhD student have also profoundly informed the shape of this book.

We acknowledge and deeply thank the digital storytelling facilitators, policy-makers, and researchers who have contributed to the conversations shared in this book by being interviewed. In particular, we would like to thank: staff at the Dementia Centre at Stirling University and the South Australian and Northern Territory Dementia Training Study Centre; Sarah Puntoni, Anna Tee, and colleagues in the 1000 Lives project; Lisa Heledd Jones of Storyworks; Professor Maggie Kirk and Karen Lewis from the University of South Wales; Pip Hardy and Tony Sumner from Pilgrim's Progress; Amy Hill from Silence Speaks; Donna McDonald of Griffith University; Holly Miller of ActionAid

Australia; Marilyn Casley of Griffith University; Cheryl Matthews of the Logan City Library; Beth Cross of the Institute for Youth and Community Research and School of Education at the University of West of Scotland; Jeanne Battello of Handicap International; and those who wish to remain anonymous.

We acknowledge and thank Connie Allen for her invaluable and extremely timely editing work on this book. Interviews and fieldwork for the book were supported by Macquarie University's Outside Studies Programme and a Macquarie University Faculty of Arts Learning and Teaching Research Grant, while essential writing time was enabled by the Macquarie University Faculty of Arts Mid-Career Fellowship. We also warmly thank the Queensland Conservatorium Research Centre and the Health Group at Griffith University for publications and research funding to support our preparation of this book.

We acknowledge and thank Professor Lesley Chenoweth AO and all current and former staff and participants in the 1000 Voices Disability Life Stories project, which gave us additional motivation to pursue many of the topics covered in this book.

Finally, we would like to acknowledge and thank our family and friends for their unflagging support over the years in which this book was conceived, researched, and written.

Abbreviations

BAs	Ban Advocates
CDS	Centre for Digital Storytelling
CMC	Cluster Munition Coalition
ICBL	International Campaign to Ban Landmines
NDIS	National Disability Insurance Scheme (Australia)
NHS	National Health Service (United Kingdom)
SDOH	Social determinants of health
UK	United Kingdom
UN	United Nations

1   Introduction

The idea that people telling stories about their own experiences of ill-health, treatment, and well-being might powerfully change health outcomes is, in some ways, revolutionary. Valuing stories involves questioning the primacy of quantitative evidence about health outcomes and treatments, and potentially disrupting biomedical concepts of illness and well-being. Paying attention to individual experiences of what makes people feel better or worse up-ends hierarchies of expertise. Attending to people's stories about their own embodied experience of well-being or care shifts perceptions that doctors, nurses, or public health officials are the people who know best about ill-health. Listening to the voices of people with personal experience of disablement and marginalisation also responds to the radical demands of the disability movement that there should be "nothing about us without us". The promise of stories as a tool for social transformation and social justice, then, is a compelling one.

Over the last twenty years, digital storytelling practitioners, health workers and educators, self-advocates, and community groups, excited by this promise, have worked with storytellers to try to enhance health and well-being. Much of what has been written about digital storytelling focuses on the collection of stories and the value to the storyteller of participating in the storytelling process. However, a few organisations – like the US Storycenter's Silence Speaks and the UK's Patient Voices – have built up a wealth of experience of not just gathering stories but using them to prompt professional learning and improvement in clinical service provision and community health. The work of these organisations has underscored the importance not only of people *telling* stories about their experiences of health and care, but of health professionals and policymakers *listening* to these experiences. It is this listening – how to prompt it and the complexities of achieving it – that is at the centre of this book.

Our first purpose in writing this book is to map some of the diverse ways in which stories of lived experience have been used to prompt listening, learning, and change in health and social policy settings internationally. Finding case studies in which the potential of stories to prompt change is practically explored, rather than just gestured towards, hasn't always been easy. We suspect there are many tales of listening to be told by digital storytelling practitioners – workshop facilitators, teachers, community health workers, or advocates – that simply never make it into print. Those with the practical expertise of making listening happen are often not those required to publish about it. Likewise, as we discuss in Chapter two, the unseen "dirty laundry" of what happens to digital stories after initial project funding runs out is not necessarily the sort of tale that funders or institutional sponsors are willing to tell or want to hear. To try to open up this important terrain, we have chosen case studies that offer a complex and honest view of listening to digital stories across a range of health and social policy settings.

In discussing the complexity of promoting listening across a range of health and social policy settings we respond to Nick Couldry's (2008) call to explore the conditions under which digital stories can be "exchanged, referred to, treated as a resource and given recognition and authority" (p. 388). Our particular aim is to unveil both the complexity and current reality of undertaking these tasks, all of which can be conceptualised as part of listening. As Jean Burgess (2006) has suggested, there is a pressing need to "understand and practically engage with the full diversity of existing and emerging media contexts in which [digital stories] are, or are not, being heard" (p. 212). Our hope is that this book will begin to map the range of contexts in which digital storytelling in a variety of forms has been used as a medium for communicating lived experience in the domain of health and social policy.

To achieve this we have also sought out practitioners and researchers who have engaged with the "nitty gritty" of getting health professionals and policy-makers to listen to others' stories. In the chapters that follow, we investigate the ways that digital stories have been listened to and learned from in professional education (Chapter three); primary and acute health care (Chapter four); community and place-based health (Chapter five); and advocacy and policymaking (Chapter six). In moving across these contexts, we shift from the individual and interpersonal level – the micro-level – at which listening to stories is often discussed, through to listening at the level of organisation and community, and finally to listening at the macro-level of national and international policymaking. In moving across these levels of analysis we aim to acknowledge the fundamental social determinants of health, as well as the role of individual health professionals and particular clinical encounters in shaping the experience of well-being.

Our cartography of this diverse terrain has required framing digital storytelling in a range of sometimes quite disparate disciplinary perspectives, from media studies and cultural theory to the sociology of health. We have also drawn on debates around health care, human services, community development, and health promotion, which accounts for our focus on both health and social policy. In our collaboration as a writing team, we often encountered surprising convergences between arguments and concepts across disciplines, and we have attempted to put similar ideas side by side. At other times, moving from one discipline to another uncovered quite disparate foundational assumptions – often unnoticed or unquestioned in previous studies and literature – that we have wrangled with and unpacked as we have moved along together.

Our second purpose with this book is to understand and theorise current listening practice. We remain passionate about the value of digital stories as a tool for social justice. However, we aim to discuss practices around listening to digital stories in a way that moves beyond idealistic visions of democratising possibilities. We will explore the complexity of listening to digital stories, and the challenges of creating occasions for listening to those stories. We have, less than we hoped, been able to access the experiences of what we might call "end users" of digital stories – although what constitutes "end use" is open to question and debate. In our search to understand how digital stories might be used to improve health and well-being, we have found ourselves talking most often to what we have called here "listening brokers", people who work to create occasions for listening to stories around health and social policy. In mapping dimensions of listening, we have relied on accounts of listening from people who were there when it happened – storytelling facilitators, patient experience managers, teachers and trainers, advocates and lobbyists. The people we have spoken to aim to encourage listening and sometimes have the power to shape circumstances in which listening happens: creating an atmosphere in a workshop, scaffolding a learning event, building routines and networks in an organisation, planning an advocacy initiative, or building a website. We want to frame these activities as anticipating, planning for, imagining, and co-constructing listening.

In pulling together this book, we undertook twenty-three interviews with practitioners in Australia, the United States (US), and the United Kingdom (UK). Against the backdrop of the academic research on digital storytelling, we've combined our own experiences of working on storytelling projects with the observations these practitioners have generously shared. We aim to distil, compare, and theorise these accounts of practice to better understand the realities, potential, and complexities of listening.

There are many handbooks of digital storytelling in print. It is our hope that this book will be useful to people who are passionate about listening to the voices of health service users. In particular, we want to provide ideas for those who aim to learn from stories of lived experience, or encourage others to learn from such stories. We would also like this book to be of value to those who have used digital storytelling in their practice and want to reflect on and extend those experiences. With this in mind, at the end of each chapter we have identified a set of "take-aways" for practitioners to think through. However, this is not a how-to book. As we track the mediation of personal stories as they move from the storyteller and storytelling workshop to lecture theatres, conference suites, board rooms, and the United Nations (UN), we aim not to simplify or codify, but to trouble and complicate existing accounts of the way life experience narratives might be used to enhance health, well-being, and social justice. But before we begin, we need to spell out what we mean by the three key terms in our title: "digital storytelling", "listening", and "health".

What do we mean by "digital storytelling"?

We use the term "digital storytelling" to refer to life-story telling in a variety of mediated forms deployed to prompt social change. Throughout this book, we discuss the important tradition of what Kelly McWilliam (2009) terms "specific" digital storytelling or what others have described as "the digital storytelling movement" or "classic" digital storytelling. Joe Lambert, founder of the StoryCenter (previously the Centre for Digital Storytelling or CDS) in Berkeley, CA, describes this approach to storytelling emerging out of the conjunction of community arts and politics:

> Corresponding directly to the extension of civil, economic, and political rights in the larger society, the community artists saw the extension of technical and aesthetic training in the arts as a civil right. They focused their efforts on providing arts access to this training to all sectors of the population who were underserved by traditional education and vocational training systems. At times the emphasis of such projects was on personal voice and the development of identity, esteem, and resilience in the individual; at other times the art making specifically addressed social conflicts and broader political issues. This legacy is at the core of our work.
>
> (Lambert, 2009)

What we will call "classic" digital stories, as produced by the CDS (now known as the StoryCenter), were three- to five-minute-long videos, comprised of images (usually personal photographs) with a first-person narration by a storyteller. Stories were normally put together during a three-day workshop, in which a group of storytellers gather, share story ideas around the "story circle", script their narrative, and pull materials together on consumer-grade software. Daniel Meadows, who was instrumental in introducing digital storytelling to the UK, characterised the themes and tone of these stories as "short, personal multimedia tales told from the heart" (Meadows, cited in Rossiter & Garcia, 2010, p. 37). The digital storytelling "movement" has attracted advocates and practitioners right around the world, and has been the subject of a range of detailed accounts (see for example, Hartley & McWilliam, 2009; Lundby, 2008; Thumim, 2009).

It would be impossible to ignore the impact of "classic" digital storytelling as a set of practices for telling autobiographical multimedia stories, and an explicit philosophy and rationale. The value of listening to digital stories has long been framed as central to the activities of digital storytellers – the StoryCenter frames its website with the strapline "listen deeply, tell stories". Several of the case studies that we focus on (e.g. the work of Silence Speaks) emerge from the StoryCenter itself or draw heavily on its methodologies and philosophies (e.g. the influential Patient Voices). However, we want to paint a broader canvas than simply the digital storytelling "movement". While practitioners in the "classic" digital storytelling tradition have made a passionate and carefully thought through argument for the differences between workshop-based participatory storytelling and other ways of generating and gathering stories (e.g. Hessler & Lambert, 2017), we want to locate this approach to digital storytelling as part of a longer history of participatory video, memoir in various forms, video diaries, photovoice, and other multimedia self-representing practices (e.g. Dovey, 2000; Matthews, 2007). In using the broader sense of the term "digital storytelling", we don't want to understate the differences between "classic" digital storytelling and other ways of eliciting personal stories, or set aside the political consequences of those differences. However, our focus on the way stories are mediated and remediated as they move to new places and listeners has suggested to us that the political meanings and outcomes of autobiographical stories can't be reduced to the process by which those stories have been generated.

Contemporary understandings of digital stories

Our conversations with people using experiential storytelling to prompt change in health care services have suggested that while the CDS model has been widely disseminated, the kinds of experiential narratives that come to be used to prompt professional learning and organisational change are diverse – often influenced by the ideas of "classic" digital storytelling, but also by other approaches to personal narrative. We want to acknowledge the diverse ways in which personal narratives have been used as resources for training aged care staff, inducting nurses, or influencing the vote of representatives at the UN not as a failure to do digital storytelling "properly", but as a response, for better or worse, to particular institutional locations, goals, and listeners. By including examples of more diverse uses of mediated autobiographical narratives we are trying to find out how personal multimedia storytelling *has* been used in health care and social service settings, not just how it *could* be used.

So what are we referring to when we speak about digital storytelling in this book? Our focus is on personal experiential stories, recorded in a variety of digital forms. Some of the case studies we will consider use video; others draw on audio recordings, photographic images, and a few digitised texts. Many of the case studies we discuss blend two or more of these forms. We do not limit our discussion of digital storytelling and listening to stories that are shared only in digital environments such as the Internet. Instead, we trace the movement of digital stories within and between online and offline settings for listening, the particular focus of Chapter two, which centres on listening environments.

Recent work has started to use the term "digital storytelling" to describe fragmented, collaboratively compiled narratives, like a Twitter feed, for example (Couldry et al., 2015). We can certainly see how online practices as diverse as Facebook status updates, in-game avatars, or micro-blogging might be conceived as forms of life-storytelling. While we will consider hyper-mediated forms of listening, particularly in Chapter two, our primary focus here is on stand-alone narratives that can be archived and thus placed side by side, led by the kinds of stories we have found being used in health and social policy settings.

What do we mean by "listening"?

Implicit in the commitment to social justice in both "specific" digital storytelling and broader participatory traditions is that those in positions of power need to listen to the experiences of others who do not typically experience that same power. In "classic" digital storytelling there is a commitment to "deep listening" as an integral element of sharing experiences in the story circle – listening by the facilitator and by participants to their peers. This listening is viewed as shaping the kinds of stories and relationships born in the story circle. Despite this interest in listening as a part of the process of telling stories and creating new forms of community, the digital storytelling literature has much less to say about the experience of listening to stories outside of this first group of attentive storyteller/listeners.

There may be a number of reasons for this lack of attention to listening outside of the story creation and telling circle. One includes a point made powerfully by Penny O'Donnell, Justine Lloyd, and Tanja Dreher (2009), that philosophies of digital storytelling have shared with much cultural theory and political activism of the last fifty years a focus on "voice". O'Donnell et al. (2009) articulate that "much of the analysis of mediated communication is modelled on a politics of expression, that is, of speaking up and out, finding a voice, making oneself heard, and so on" (p. 423).

In the past decade there has been a new attention to listening as a critical element of communication (Couldry, 2010; Dreher, 2012; Lacey, 2013; Lloyd, 2009; Thill, 2015). Listening as understood by these scholars and those they draw on – notably the work of Susan Bickford – is fundamentally political. Listening is not simply an interpersonal or individual process but one in which collective identities and inequalities of power are almost inevitably implicated. As Justine Lloyd (2009) has pointed out, there has also been a revaluing of listening in a corporate culture, but political listening seeks to mobilise change in ways that exceed the "customer service" intentions of such corporate listening (Lloyd, 2009; Macnamara, 2015). Bickford's account of listening, which mobilises the work of philosophers such as Hannah Arendt and Audre Lorde, stresses instead the dissonances – conflict, disagreements, and disjunctions – that are part of the process of political listening. She emphasises the emotional investments that are required for such listening: the need to overcome fear in order to listen, or the role of shame at one's limited understanding in prompting purposeful listening. In Bickford's formulation, listening does not require self-abnegation, the listener suppressing or denying their own point of view. Rather, this understanding views the listener's perspectives as the ground of communication, while what is said by the person to whom one listens is the figure emerging against that ground. This work moves away from more conventional understandings of speaking as active, and listening as passive (Lloyd, 2009, p. 478). Political listening is instead framed as often difficult, emotionally draining cultural work, requiring openness to others, a commitment to an ongoing engagement and, frequently, courage (Bickford, 1996; Thill, 2009, 2015; Lloyd, 2009).

Endorsing a non-audist concept of listening

Before proceeding further, we should emphasise that, despite the aural metaphor embedded in the term "listening", our interest is not in the physiological process of hearing. Many Deaf people, for example, are expert listeners, nimbly switching between modes of communication, ever vigilant about the possibility of communication breakdown and generous with their time and attention in the quest to understand what someone else has to convey. Equally, many of the stories we discuss include a visual as well as auditory or textual component. Our use of the term "listening" does not exclude consideration of the impact or importance of the visual element of these stories. Our emphasis throughout the book is on attention and attunement to personal narratives. We use the term "listening" as a complement to the widespread metaphorical use of the term "voice". "Having a voice" and "being given a voice" have long been used as phrases to refer to opportunities for agency or participation. Our use of the term "listening", then, takes up the metaphor – so familiar that its aural component often goes unnoticed – and shifts our attention to the complement of voice, that is, attention, attunement, awareness of another person's views, perspectives, or story.

Listening as mediation and transformation

Extending the work of Couldry (2008) and others (for example, Iedema, 2003; Silverstone, 1999; Sunderland, 2009), we frame the process of listening to digital stories as involving a series of processes of "mediation". We adopt Silverstone's definition of mediation as the "movement of meanings" to support our understanding of listening and mediation:

> Mediation involves the movement of meaning from one text to another, from one discourse to another, from one event to another. It involves the constant transformation of meanings, both large scale and small, significant and insignificant, as media texts and texts about media circulate in writing, in speech and audiovisual forms, and as we, individually and collectively, directly and indirectly, contribute to their production.
>
> (Silverstone, 1999, p. 13)

By emphasising the way stories are subject to intended and unintended processes of mediation we will explore the inevitable dislocations and transformations of meaning and agency that occur through listening. A core assumption of our work is that processes of listening and mediation are never neutral or wholly "controllable". Rather, they are always socially embedded, interpretive, and politically, economically, and ethically significant (Silverstone, 1999). Mediation and listening are also inevitably located within socio-historical and political trajectories and systems. Any process of mediation necessarily involves complex repeated processes of translation and resemiotisation (movement of meaning into new languages or semiotic systems), remediation (movement of meaning into new media types such as websites, reports, films, and meetings), and recontextualisation (movement of meanings into new social contexts such as education, policymaking, or service delivery). We collectively refer to the above interlinked processes as "mediation" for the purposes of this book.

Rick Iedema's (1997, 2000) work on recontextualisation in bureaucratic contexts illustrates the ways that personal meanings can become part of a series of potentially depersonalised bureaucratic processes. Meanings such as those conveyed in personal digital stories are mediated into increasingly durable artefacts, such as meeting minutes, reports, plans, buildings, and services. The consequence of these particular processes of bureaucratic recontextualisation – which are common to policymaking processes – is that increasingly durable materialities (e.g. a hospital building, service, or product) are seen to literally encapsulate the meanings and "voices" that have shaped their creation, and become resources for meaning making and lived experience in themselves (Iedema, 2000). In many cases it can be difficult to discern exactly how diverse personal stories and other forms of evidence and knowledge are (or are not) woven into the complex outcomes and materialities that then shape people's daily lives. This is a point we return to in Chapter six, as we discuss the "black box" of how digital stories are used in policymaking.

As the case studies in this book show, listening to personal digital stories in diverse health and social policy settings involves constant processes of mediation, whereby a personal story is re-presented in a way that makes it suitable to be moved, shared, and "used". The storyteller chooses ways of speaking about their experience that draw on the narrative resources, for example genres (Poletti, 2011) or "emplotments" (Frank, 1995), available to them. Consequently, even the first step of storytelling is a form of mediation that filters the range of meanings on offer for listeners to that story. The act of listening to another's story in *any* context also involves mediating movements of – at a minimum – translation, as the listener interprets the other's story and "brings it home" to their own ways of making sense of (and acting upon) that story. Sarangi (1998) observes that these acts of mediation imply *creativity* (pp. 306–307) rather than reproduction. This idea of the reframing and reproduction as being a space of loss and threat, while also being potentially generative, is one we will return to throughout the book.

As digital stories are mediated, they are often moved beyond the direct "reach" or control of the storyteller. A handwritten autobiographical narrative that enters a new medium (e.g. by being scanned and shared on a web repository) or comes to be used in a new context (e.g. policymaking) is being mediated by any number of other agents who may influence the processes and outcomes of listening. While decisions about what might be an appropriate use of a story may be controlled by storytellers themselves to some extent, more often those who control the medium through which the story moves have greater control. This applies as much to online storytelling settings as it does in policymaking and public consultation settings. The mediation lens hence helps us to problematise moral and political agency in listening processes.

Extending the notion of mediation in the specific context of personal storytelling, a number of writers working around what they have dubbed "auto/biography" have argued that stories are not simply narratives of individual storytellers, but are often solicited or "coaxed" (in the words of Smith & Watson, 2001) from storytellers by particular institutions or social settings – the appointment with the psychologist, visit to the job centre, witness statement in the courtroom, or visa application narrative (Hall & Rossmanith, 2016; Poletti, 2011; Stanley, 2002). This perspective proposes shifting from an expressivist view of life story that vests authenticity in narratives devoid of any intervention by media "experts", to one that sees experiences as organised and shaped through encounters with institutions, genres, social processes, and relationships. This approach draws heavily from feminist understandings of life narratives.

Our work here is deeply informed by this socially embedded approach to life storytelling. We emphasise that there is no "before" or "after" to processes of mediation; it is an inherent and unavoidable element of both storytelling and listening. This fundamentally shifts our perspective on the way digital stories might be used. Rather than seeing the deployment of digital stories as a potentially dangerous wresting of control of the narrative from the storyteller, a focus on auto/biography as always mediated suggests that stories come to be born in particular times and places, shaped by particular demands to speak about some topics in particular languages, and remain silent about others. In other words, auto/biographical narratives never have an "authentic", "unmediated" innocence to lose. A storyteller stepping into a boardroom to talk about their experiences of an ambulance service is going to have their story shaped by the languages, listeners, and spaces around them. A story pulled together from personal photos with a voice-over, in the "specific" digital storytelling tradition is also shaped by the story circle sharing process, facilitator experience, and affordances of video and computer technology. Our focus, then, is on the ways in which particular personal stories might move through new spaces and gather new listeners. How does this mediation shift the ways these stories work? Where might stories, spaces, and listeners collectively enable social change? How are these things happening in practice in our selected case studies?

As O'Donnell et al. (2009) point out, understanding listening in behaviourist terms doesn't reflect the complexity of the process. While the language of "outcomes" and "impact" has come to be very influential in the types of institutions that have looked to storytellers as agents of transformation – health systems, for example – we don't want to be reductive about listening.

Demonstrable changes in institutions and practices might mark out successful moments of listening, but an absence of such changes may not indicate that listening hasn't occurred. Social change can be non-linear and incremental, and we wanted to remain open to this kind of complexity.

What do we mean by "health"?

The way we have organised this book – moving from a focus on listening as individuals and organisations, to local communities and international policy-making settings – speaks to the way we understand health and what shapes it. While we start by considering individual encounters in the clinical context of primary health, we move "upstream" and outwards to consider the way attention to personal stories might help change the meso- and macro-level social and environmental determinants of health and well-being, such as health and social policy, and the environment (see Schulz & Northridge, 2004). Activists and researchers taking this approach seek to focus on a radical reformulation of the concept of preventative health that involves alleviating the social and economic inequalities, social exclusion, and marginalisation that lead to health inequalities, rather than focusing on acute care after people have developed illness and ailments (see for example, Marmot & Bell, 2012; Marmot, 2005; Schulz & Northridge, 2004).

International policymakers have long acknowledged the role of social, political, environmental, and cultural factors in shaping individual experiences of health and well-being, reflecting the World Health Organization's (WHO, 1948) long-standing definition of "health" as a "state of complete physical, mental and social well-being and not merely the absence of disease or infirmity" (n.p.). International agreements such as the *Declaration of Alma-Ata* (WHO, 1978), the *Global Strategy for Health for All by the Year 2000* (WHO, 1981), the *Ottawa Charter for Health Promotion* (WHO, 1986), and the *Jakarta Declaration on Leading Health Promotion into the 21st Century* (WHO, 1997) all reinforce that social, environmental, and economic factors and inequalities are the primary determinants of individuals' health and well-being. By adopting a social determinants model of health, we expand our conversation on digital stories in health and social policy to include a politicised reading of health and well-being. This political and social view of health and well-being matches the politicised understandings of "voice", marginalisation, and social justice that underpin much digital storytelling activity.

Storytelling, self-determination, and the social determinants of health

A key message of the *Ottawa Charter for Health Promotion* is that citizens must be able to exercise self-determination in relation to their own health and well-being:

> Health promotion is the process of enabling people to increase control over, and to improve, their health. To reach a state of complete physical,

mental and social well-being, an individual or group must be able to identify and to realize aspirations, to satisfy needs, and to change or cope with the environment. Health is, therefore, seen as a resource for everyday life, not the objective of living. Health is a positive concept emphasizing social and personal resources, as well as physical capacities. Therefore, health promotion is not just the responsibility of the health sector, but goes beyond healthy life-styles to well-being.

(WHO, 1986, n.p.)

This awareness of the importance of self-determination underpins many health-related storytelling projects in community or neighbourhood-based storytelling. Many of these projects aim to use storytelling to: (1) unveil and understand the complexity of service user and citizen experiences of health and well-being, and (2) engage storytellers in shared decision making or con-sultation activities.

These aims for self-determination and health, converge with demands by disability and other activists to be actively involved in all steps of decision making ("nothing about us without us"), not just "consulted" in decisions relating to their own welfare and needs (see Charlton, 1998). A focus on the social determinants of health aligns with the disability movement's critique of biomedical models of disability, and the preference for social models that position disability as politicised difference rather than medical defect. At its broadest level, disability self-advocates and others are demanding a radical reconfiguration of oppressive ways of seeing, being, and acting that result in the devaluing, social exclusion, and marginalisation of some groups of people, and consequent adverse social, health, and well-being outcomes. In the more specific context of health care delivery, consumers are asking to be listened to in relation to their personal experiences of health care service delivery. While these political movements and imperatives have often been viewed as claiming "a voice" in the bureaucracies and processes that shape people's lives, they are also demands that powerful people – professionals, policymakers, and bureaucrats – are starting to respond to through being able to listen to those voices.

Outline of the chapters

Chapter two provides a platform for later chapters by surveying con-temporary listening environments that shape listening. We also introduce four "meta-oratory" roles that people who influence listening environments have in relation to the way that stories are presented and listened to. These include the roles of the story curator, broker, host, and caretaker. Taking these meta-oratory roles into account, we then describe case studies of major offline and online listening environments under three categories: listening occasions, online digital infrastructures, and social media.

Chapter three examines applications of digital storytelling in professional health education. This context emphasises the impact that listening to digital stories has on health care service providers who, in turn, directly shape health care experiences for service consumers or patients. Hence this chapter explores individual and interpersonal applications of digital story listening. The practice case study for this chapter focuses on listening to digital stories in dementia care education.

Chapter four provides an in-depth account of the ways that digital stories are being listened to in primary and acute care settings such as hospitals. This chapter examines the ways that health and social care systems are being set up to listen institutionally to patient stories. These systems function as significant meso-level determinants of health. Because a lot of this work is already being done in the UK, we focus on two UK case studies: a Welsh listening project called 1000 Lives Plus and the well-known Patient Stories project.

Chapter five moves away from clinical health practice and policy to examine digital storytelling and listening in meso-level community and place-based health promotion settings. We draw on interdisciplinary theory and literature to emphasise the importance and realities of embodied, emplaced, and ecological approaches to listening. This chapter features a case study of a digital storytelling project with Grade five children who researched and documented happy, healthy local places as part of a district-wide health coalition research project.

Chapter six extends our conversation to include national and international policymaking settings that shape the macro social determinants of health and well-being. We review the existing academic literature to determine the degree to which digital stories are being listened and responded to by policy and decision makers. We then supplement this review with case studies of the National Disability Insurance Scheme (NDIS) in Australia and the international Ban Advocates project led by Handicap International in Belgium.

Chapter seven provides a summary and conclusion for the book, and emphasises the major learnings and themes from across the various contexts explored in earlier chapters.

References

Bickford, S. (1996). *The Dissonance of Democracy: Listening, Conflict and Citizenship.* Ithaca, NY: Cornell University Press.

Burgess, J. E. (2006). Hearing ordinary voices: Cultural studies, vernacular creativity and digital storytelling. *Continuum: Journal of Media and Cultural Studies, 20*(2), 201–214.

Charlton, J. I. (1998). *Nothing about Us without Us: Disability Oppression and Empowerment.* Berkeley: University of California Press.

Couldry, N. (2008). Mediatization or mediation? Alternative understandings of the emergent space of digital storytelling. *New Media and Society, 10*(3), 373–391. doi: 10.1177/1461444808089414

Couldry, N. (2010). *Why Voice Matters: Culture and Politics after Neoliberalism.* London: Sage.

Couldry, N., McDonald, R., Stephansen, H., Clark, W., Dickens, L., & Fotopoulou, A. (2015). Constructing a digital story circle: Digital infrastructure and mutual recognition. *International Journal of Cultural Studies, 18*(5), 501–517.

Dovey, J. (2000). *Freakshow: First Person Media and Factual Television.* London: Pluto Press.

Dreher, T. (2012) A partial promise of voice? Digital storytelling and the limits of listening. *Media International Australia, 142,* 157–166.

Frank, A. W. (1995). *The Wounded Storyteller: Body, Illness and Ethics.* Chicago, IL: University of Chicago Press.

Hall, M., & Rossmanith, K. (2016). Imposed stories: Prisoner self-narratives in the criminal justice system. *International Journal for Crime, Justice and Social Democracy, 5*(1). doi: http://dx.doi.org/10.5204/ijcjsd.v5i1.284

Hartley, J., & McWilliam, K. (Eds.) (2009). *Story Circle: Digital Storytelling around the World.* Chichester: Wiley Blackwell.

Hessler, B., & Lambert, J. (2017, forthcoming). Threshold concepts of digital storytelling: Naming what we know about storywork. In Y. Nordkvelle, G. Jamissen, P. Hardy, & H. Pleasants (Eds.), *Digital Storytelling in Higher Education: International Perspectives.* Melbourne: Palgrave Macmillan.

Iedema, R. (1997). The language of administration. Organizing human activity in formal institutions. In F. Christie & J. R. Martin (Eds.), *Genre and Institutions. Social Processes in the Workplace and School* (pp. 40–72). London: Continuum.

Iedema, R. (2000). Bureaucratic planning and resemiotisation. In E. Ventola (Ed.), *Discourse and Community. Doing Functional Linguistics* (pp. 47–70). Tubingen: Gunter Narr Verlag Tumingen.

Iedema, R. (2003). Multimodality, resemiotization: Extending the analysis of discourse as multi-semiotic practice. *Visual Communication, 2*(1), 29–57.

Lacey, K. (2013). *Listening Publics: The Politics and Experience of Listening in the Media Age.* Cambridge: Polity Press.

Lambert, J. (2009). The history of CDS. A short story behind the stories by CDS founder Joe Lambert. *Centre for Digital Storytelling* [website]. Retrieved from http://www.storycenter.org/press/

Lloyd, J. (2009). The listening cure. *Continuum: Journal of Media and Cultural Studies, 23*(4), 477–487.

Lundby, K. (Ed.). (2008). *Digital Storytelling, Mediatized Stories: Self-Representations in New Media.* New York: Peter Lang.

Macnamara, J. (2015). *Organizational Listening. The Missing Essential in Public Communication.* New York: Peter Lang.

McWilliam, K. (2009). The global diffusion of a community media practice: Digital storytelling online. In J. Hartley & K. McWilliam (Eds.), *Story Circle: Digital Storytelling around the World* (pp. 37–76). Chichester: Wiley Blackwell.

Marmot, M. (2005). Social determinants of health inequalities. *The Lancet, 365*(9464), 1099–1104.

Marmot, M., & Bell, R. (2012). Fair society, healthy lives. *Public Health, 126,* S4–S10.

Matthews, N. (2007). Confessions to a new public: Video Nation shorts. *Media, Culture and Society, 29*(3), 435–448. doi: 10.1177/0163443707076184

O'Donnell, P., Lloyd, J., & Dreher, T. (2009). Listening, pathbuilding and continuations: A research agenda for the analysis of listening. *Continuum: Journal of Media and Cultural Studies, 23*(4), 423–439.

Poletti, A. (2011). Coaxing an intimate public: Life narrative in digital storytelling. *Continuum: Journal of Media and Cultural Studies* , *25*(1), 73–83.

Rossiter, M., & Garcia, P. A. (2010). Digital storytelling: A new player on the narrative field. *New Directions for Adult and Continuing Education*, *126*, 37–48. doi: 10.1002/ace.370

Sarangi, S. (1998). Rethinking recontextualisation in professional discourse studies: An epilogue. *Text*, *18*(2), 301–318.

Schulz, A., & Northridge, M. E. (2004). Social determinants of health: Implications for environmental health promotion. *Health Education & Behavior*, *31*(4), 455–471.

Silverstone, R. (1999). *Why Study the Media?* Thousand Oaks, CA: Sage.

Smith, S., & Watson, J. 2001. *Reading Autobiography: A Guide for Interpreting Life Narratives*. Minneapolis and London: University of Minnesota Press.

Stanley, L. (2002). From 'self-made women' to 'women's made-selves': Audit selves, simulation and surveillance in the rise of the public woman. In T. Cosslett, C. Lury, & P. Summerfield (Eds.), *Feminism and Autobiography: Text, Theories, Methods* (pp. 40–60). London: Routledge.

Sunderland, N. (2009). Virtuous or vicious? Agency and representation in biotechnology's virtuous cycle. *Journal of Technical Writing and Communication*, *39*(4), 381–400.

Thill, C. (2009). Courageous listening, responsibility for the other and the Northern Territory Intervention. *Continuum: Journal of Media and Cultural Studies*, *23*(4), 537–548.

Thill, C. (2015). Listening for policy change: How the voices of disabled people shaped Australia's National Disability Insurance Scheme. *Disability and Society*, *30*(1), 15–28.

Thumim, N. (2009). 'Everyone has a story to tell'. Mediation and self-representation in two UK institutions. *International Journal of Cultural Studies*, *12*(6), 617–638.

WHO (1948). *WHO Definition of Health*. Retrieved from http://www.who.int/about/definition/en/print.html

WHO (1978). *Declaration of Alma-Ata*. Retrieved from http://www.who.int/publications/almaata_declaration_en.pdf

WHO (1981). *Global Strategy for Health for All by the Year 2000*. Retrieved from http://www.un-documents.net/a36r43.htm

WHO (1986). *Ottawa Charter for Health Promotion*. Retrieved from http://www.who.int/healthpromotion/conferences/previous/ottawa/en/

WHO (1997). *Jakarta Declaration on Leading Health Promotion into the 21st Century*. Retrieved from http://www.who.int/healthpromotion/conferences/previous/jakarta/declaration/en/

2 Listening environments

A starting point for this book is that digital stories, in all of their diverse forms, are inevitably mediated and transformed as they move from story-tellers to listeners. This chapter explores the fundamental and practical ways that diverse environments for listening shape the way that stories are moved and transformed and, as a result, the way that listeners might experience and make sense of digital stories. We will explore both online and offline environments for listening across three categories. First, we discuss offline social occasions for listening such as story circles, project launches, or exhibitions that are featured in much of the existing digital storytelling literature. Second, we examine bespoke infrastructures for story listening such as online repositories of digital stories. Finally, we examine listening via more generalised social media platforms such as YouTube, blogs, and Facebook. These diverse environments constitute meta-contexts for listening across the health and social policy contexts and activities we explore in subsequent chapters of this book. We remind readers at the outset that these listening environments are not "neutral" or devoid of political and cultural significance. We observe that if storytellers are orators, listening environments and the people who create and maintain them are "meta-orators": orienting, often seamlessly and invisibly, the way people find, understand, listen to, and attend to personal stories.

Occasions of listening

Much of the existing work on listening in academic writing around digital storytelling has focused on what we might call "occasions" of listening during story creation and after stories are complete. These can include workshop processes such as story circles that are used to promote dialogic listening and storytelling, community building, and other public events such as story exhibitions. A significant feature of these listening occasions is their ephemerality when contrasted to longer-lasting listening environments such as online repositories of stories. A second feature of such listening occasions is that they are typically conducted in person in shared, physical, and geographical time and space rather than asynchronously online. We will explore some of the dynamics of listening during these occasions below.

Story circles and workshops

Most published work on listening in "classic" digital storytelling contexts has focused on the way listening happens in the story circle, as storytellers share ideas about their stories with one another (Lambert cited in Wang, 2013, p. 151; see also Alexandra, 2015; Clarke, 2014; Thumim, 2007). In the story circle, facilitators ask storytellers to pay careful attention to the experiences of others who are also participating in workshops, which characterises this style of digital storytelling. These processes are central to the Center for Digital Storytelling (CDS, now known as "Storycenter") process. The website for Storycenter is subtitled "Listen deeply, tell stories", which underscores the idea that listening is both necessary before and profoundly linked to telling your own story. Brooke Hessler and Joe Lambert (2017) have described listening in classic digital storytelling as embodied, cognitive, and metacognitive "generative listening", as "both an ethic and a craft" essential to the storytelling process. The importance of creating a respectful and empathetic listening environment and sense of community in the Storycenter story circles has been discussed in many accounts of the digital storytelling workshop (see for example, Hardy & Sumner, 2014; Lambert, 2009; Hessler & Lambert, 2017). Emerging from radical pedagogy and community education movements, participatory workshop-based digital storytelling is underpinned by a dialogic understanding of knowledge production (Polk, 2010) which stresses both speaking and listening.

In addition to being shaped by storytelling peers, listening in the story circle is also explicitly scaffolded by storytelling facilitators. As Pip Hardy of Pilgrim Projects, who has facilitated hundreds of digital stories, comments:

> we give [participants] quite specific instructions about how to listen, and then how to offer constructive feedback … We encourage them to listen for what's not said as well as for what is said … listen for the silence … at some point, you see their eyes fill with tears, and their voice cracks. Then you know that you're going to get the real story.
>
> (personal communication)

Listening carefully to others' narratives in the story circle helps participants reflect on the story they want to tell themselves, to think about the elements of a good story, and to identify the right kind of language to use. Reflective listening also allows participants to hone the craft of storytelling. However, co-founder of Pilgrim Projects, Tony Sumner, articulates other ways that listening in the story circle can function:

> the group process is very powerful … because of the groups we engage with, we very often get someone who is incandescently angry about the treatment … that a relative or a loved one has had, or the lack of it … One case in particular comes to mind where there was a lovely guy who was a carer for his wife. He was there with a group of other carers as

well. … they were effectively saying, "You know … if you can't tell this in such a way that people will listen to it, your message is not going to get anywhere. No-one will listen." … He didn't tone his story down, but he was then able to understand that he needed to reshape it in such a way that people would listen to it … listening helps people to make their stories more listenable…

(personal communication)

Tony's account highlights that listeners in the story circle help to shape stories, at least for Pip and Tony's storytellers, who nearly always come to workshops with the aim of changing health practices and services. Even at this earliest moment in the creation of stories, considerations about the listening environment, who will be listening to the finished story, and how stories will be received come into play.

Amy Hill from StoryCenter's Silence Speaks program also emphasises that considerations around the ultimate audience, at least for her work, often shape the way storytellers are recruited to the workshop and the prompt questions that are used to help storytelling construct a narrative:

One of the things we will very often do is work with our partner organisations to come up with very, very specific story prompts or themes that provide a starting point or umbrella for the workshop. So it's not like "Hey! We're going to do a workshop with HIV positive people. Come and tell your story." Instead, we say "This project is focused on stigma within this community. These are the hoped for audiences, these are the pressing issues. Given all that, tell a story about a moment when …" "The moment when" part is all geared towards fulfilling the objectives of the sponsoring organization. And we even do that when there's a policy agenda. We'll say, "What is your policy objective? What are the policies that you're advocating for?" Then let us know what those are and then we can craft story prompts and themes that will support people in addressing those points. That's woven across all of our public health work.

(personal communication)

Hill stresses that the skill of the facilitator is making sure that storytellers "feel really good about it and feel a sense of ownership and pride" at the same time as the partner organisations' aims are met. Karen Lewis, one of the producers of the groundbreaking BBC *Capture Wales* project, which drew heavily on the CDS participatory workshop model, makes a similar point. She argues that facilitators, listening to stories in the story circle during the many workshops around Wales, had to "listen out for stories that would work as broadcast material, whilst honouring the intent of the teller" (Lewis & Matthews, 2017). Each of these examples from experienced practitioners using a participatory workshop format to produce "classic" digital stories points out the way that right from the very moment where stories are conceived, there is an anticipation by commissioning organisations, facil-itators, and even members of the story circle of the kinds of listeners that might ultimately hear the story. So while much of the attention to listening in participatory workshop settings has been to listening within the story circle, the boundaries between the story circle and other listening contexts are more porous than we might think.

Celebratory and public events

A second space for listening to personal stories in digital storytelling projects is often the celebratory screening or public launch, a common feature of com-munity digital storytelling projects. Such occasions usually include storytellers, their family and friends, and often members of the wider community, sometimes including community leaders, politicians, public servants, and other "VIPs" (Dreher, 2012; Gubrium, Hill, & Flicker, 2014; Lewis & Matthews, 2017). These events often focus on celebration of the individual storyteller and have a "noticeable 'buzz' … a 'feel good mood'", that may, as Tanja Dreher (2012) points out, undermine a more serious political engagement with the issues raised in some stories. One of the digital story facilitators we spoke to during our preparation for this book referred to smaller, localised listening environments such as a public launch or exhibition as "preaching to the converted". Often the audiences are there because they want to support the intentions of either the storytellers, their stories, or both. While we are interested in how digital stories can shape and reshape fundamental macro- and meso-level social determinants of health in this book, we don't want to dismiss the potential power of local, interpersonal, "micro"-level transformations that can occur through different listening environments. Storytelling in intimate spaces and moments can be the glue that cements a new relationship or reinforces an advocacy network's resolve to continue their work. It can also be the space that provides a fertile bed for larger dreams to germinate. Nonetheless, as Tanja Dreher (2012) suggests, the evidence of such screenings impacting on the VIPs in attendance, let alone wider, privileged audiences, remains patchy.

Strategic formal listening occasions

In addition to the public celebratory events discussed above, digital stories can be shown at more formal and strategic occasions such as board meetings, conventions, and conferences. In these cases there is typically an emphasis on those who are listening developing some form of action or response to the stories. These occasions often include an exhibition of stories accompanied by participation by storytellers "in person" alongside storytelling facilitators or other listening brokers. Because the focus is on influencing decision making in these contexts there can often be a desire for immediate response or uptake of the knowledge and experience conveyed in digital stories (see for example, Sunderland, Bristed, Gudes, Boddy, & Da Silva, 2012).

Learning occasions

As we will discuss in some detail in Chapter three, another key space for listening to digital stories is for learning. While our discussion of processes of listening to personal multimedia stories in the next chapter focuses on professional learning by health workers, digital stories have been widely used, notably by Hill's Silence Speaks, in community and public education settings. In comparison to listening in the story circle, much less has been written about the listening that takes place when digital stories are used in training contexts. However, some organisations, including Silence Speaks, have developed resources and strategies that support and frame listening in training and education.

Temporal and spatial limits of listening occasions

The types of listening occasions we have discussed above are by definition ephemeral and located, unless there is some form of remediation and recording of the event through, for example, a mini-documentary or photos and testimonials about the event. They are also typically contained to a specific geographical place which greatly determines who participates in the listening event. There are good reasons why accounts of listening to digital stories tend to focus on the period during storytelling workshops or immediately after stories are composed. Many digital storytelling projects are based on short-term grant funding and often research around them must be squeezed into the three years of a researcher's PhD, or an even shorter period of fieldwork. As Amy Hill of Silence Speaks and Mandy Rose of *Capture Wales* remind us, there is rarely funding for follow-up research on the impact of stories. These pragmatic factors have had an impact on the types of listening environment that have been discussed in the existing literatures. A focus on listening by participants in storytelling workshops (Alexandra, 2015) or on community screenings (Dreher, 2012) has produced theoretically and empirically rich accounts of listening. Given the accessibility of participants – especially marginalised speakers like Alexander's refugees to Ireland – there is an unmissable opportunity to garner rich accounts of listening in these contexts.

Beyond the listening occasion: what happens next?

Since much of the existing work on listening in the realm of digital storytelling has focused on immediate and planned occasions of listening, we want to move beyond these occasions to focus on longer-term listening to digital stories, and the infrastructures and environments that might facilitate such listening. In doing so, we are responding to calls by a number of scholars for a longer-term perspective on the process and legacies of storytelling (Burgess, 2006; Dreher, 2012). In emphasising the complexity of circulating digital stories "after the fact" of digital storytelling projects themselves, we are also lifting the veil on the not-always-elevating afterlives of digital storytelling projects. We have found few accounts of listening that reflect on "what happens after" in the published literature (for an exception, see Gubrium et al., 2014). As well as the methodological challenges of finding what happens to stories after their launch, there are potentially high political and institutional stakes in acknowledging the virtual and not so virtual scrapheap where many digital storytelling projects end up. For example, with short-term funding of projects comes the requirement to bid for repeated tranches of funding and to report on the impact and outcome of existing projects. In work with marginalised and vulnerable communities there can also be a compelling pressure to "talk up" the continuing benefits and impact of participatory storytelling, and a reluctance to disclose any difficulties and obstacles (Copeland & Miskelly, 2010; Dush, 2013). As Nancy Thumim's (2007) account of the uses of digital storytelling by institutions like museums and broadcasters has pointed out, digital storytelling projects are engaged with democratising and social justice language, but the benefits to institutions of the appearance of reaching out, being inclusive, accessible, and transparent – what Harrison and Mort (1998) describe as "playing the user card" – should not be underestimated (see also Mitchell, 2015).

The above are all powerful reasons for individual researchers and institutions to focus on the immediate and proximal benefits to participants and struggle a little less hard than they might to give an account of how the outcomes of stories are stored, managed, circulated, publicised, used, and remembered in the longer run. Our interviews with practitioners involved in the long-term caretaking of digital story collections have underlined that insufficient time or resources often means that decisions about what happens next to stories are often made pragmatically and on the fly rather than being carefully thought through. However serendipitous their origins, the listening environments that stories move into after the funded project concludes are of great interest.

Consequently here we also focus on some of the listening environments, or listening infrastructures, that have been developed to prompt listening over the longer term. Rather than just focus on isolated listening occasions, we want to explore the complexities of listening and agency when stories are mediated from listening occasions into longer-lasting listening infrastructures and social media and sometimes back again.

Case study: A story of expected and unexpected mediations over time between listening environments

The following case study derives from our own storytelling facilitation projects and related research during a photovoice storytelling project in Australia. The data for the case study has been anonymised from the original research project within the parameters of the original ethics consent arrangements approved by Griffith University. The case study also draws on an interview conducted in 2016 with one of the project partners and the authors' own reflections and records between 2010 and 2016. The 2016 interview was conducted under a new ethics protocol approved by Griffith University. This case study was circulated to three project stakeholders for comment prior to publication. All storytellers in this project requested to remain anonymous in the original consent procedures undertaken for the project.

In 2010 a small group of non-government and government organisations and one university in Australia came together to run a photovoice project. The purpose of the project was to "visualise health" by documenting local social determinants of health and well-being for local residents in a rural town that experienced significant socio-economic disadvantage and chronic illness. A professional photographer was hired to work with local community members to create photovoice stories about their lives and what made them "happy" and "healthy". The photographer worked using a community development approach that privileged Australian Aboriginal ways of working, community leadership, consensus decision making, and immersive partnership building between the participants and the non-government organisations that were involved. On many occasions this meant that the photographer had to challenge and reject institutional and bureaucratised ways of working requested or required by the university. The photographer's work resulted in four organisations entering into a partnership to facilitate and conduct the project. This included the university where she was employed, a local Aboriginal housing organisation, a local human services organisation, and a district health coalition funded by the state health department. This was an extremely valuable and powerful project that was heralded by and a credit to the partners and participants involved. Without wanting to detract from the outcomes of the original project, this case study focuses on the largely unplanned afterlives of the project stories specifically to illuminate the complex and overlapping systems, institutions, and environments that shape listening. Thus this case study offers a "behind the scenes" look at aspects of digital storytelling that are rarely discussed in the existing academic literature.

All participants in the storytelling project were recruited via the human services organisation and the Aboriginal housing organisation involved in the project. The project was processed through the university's human research ethics committee after extensive consultation on the ethical consent processes with partners. Each individual storyteller then received written consent information prior to agreeing to participate in the project. The consent information included information that the resulting photovoice stories may be reused in online and other publications and exhibitions for not-for-profit purposes. All storytellers requested to remain anonymous in the research and any subsequent publications about the project, which has shaped the way that this case study is presented. The project also included a significant number of Aboriginal storytellers, which enhanced the need to provide participant and partner organisation control over the dissemination of stories given the abusive colonial history of Australia which had, for centuries, dehumanised and exploited Aboriginal culture, story, and peoples.

The first curated listening "occasion" for the project stories was a public art gallery exhibition of printed photos with small interview excerpts printed on cards next to the photos in June 2011. This event was closely negotiated by the photographer with storytelling participants and project partners. At the exhibition launch the Chair of the Aboriginal housing partner organisation said that he thought the photographer was one of the "best community development workers" he had ever met due to her engagement with the diverse groups and individuals. Storytellers and project partners attended the exhibition's opening and many attendees remarked that it felt like a community-run and -owned event. The audience for this event was comprised primarily of the participants and partners and their family members and friends. It also included some of the local community members. While the gallery space was enduring, the exhibition itself was relatively short-lived and only lasted for one week after the official opening. Project partners reported that they felt very emotional at the event and that the participant stories had reinforced to them the importance of certain community services, for example, the provision of human services and social work in the local caravan park. This was an example of immediate uptake of stories in the context of practice by partner representatives. It was also an example of how what some might believe to be "preaching to the converted" can lead to very positive and affirming "re-learning" or reinvigorating of localised social justice spirit.

The second deliberate and negotiated listening occasion for the project partners included a series of community health partnership network meetings which a project researcher attended but the photographer, storytellers, and project partners did not. This environment represented a second movement of meanings away from the original storytellers that was enabled via the separation of stories from their tellers by recording in digital form. The structure of the meetings and the broader community health partnership within which the project took place created an environment for listening to, interpreting, and responding to the stories that did not include any of the original project participants or decision makers. The researcher presented a series of photos from participant stories as a PowerPoint presentation along with textual excerpts from their accompanying interviews. This remediation and recontextualisation of the stories resulted in immediate uptake of information from the stories by members of the network coalition Board. These board members resolved to inquire into drug and alcohol services that were provided in the area and advocate for services to be provided if they were not already accessible. The researcher had deliberately not included music in the presentation to the Board in an attempt to reduce the impression that she was layering emotional meaning over the photo stories and trying to elicit emotive responses from decision makers. Interestingly the acting manager of the Board said after the meeting: "we need to show this to the [health department] executive! We should include some moving music behind the images to really enhance the impact!" In this case the acting manager was acting as a new "host" for the stories to be shared and listened to in the context of the meetings he chaired. This was different to the curatorial role that the photographer had originally taken in compiling and selecting the range of stories to be included and the project partner representatives' roles in caretaking the resulting stories.

While the photographer's official role as project facilitator and exhibition curator had ended after the exhibition in mid-2011 when funding ran out for the project, the researcher and other partner representatives remained as "caretakers" of the stories, which were handed to all project partners on a DVD at the conclusion of the final meeting. The caretakers attempted to continue the project in the manner that the photographer had agreed with the storytellers and partners. For example, several members of the District Health Coalition who were not directly involved in the project had requested access to the story files so that they could be used to promote the activity of the Health Coalition. The researcher remembers participating in a meeting where she initially refused access to the digital story files (i.e. photovoice stories and interviews) for local council members based, again, on the agreements that had been made between the photographer, the storytelling participants, and the partner organisations. This was not based on a lack of trust or lack of faith in the good intentions between the people involved but, rather, a desire to "stay true" to the agreements the photographer had made with the original storytellers and partner organisations. Perhaps ironically, this impulse to "stay true" to the original intentions and intended audiences had hindered opportunities to share the stories for potential social justice and policymaking applications.

The researcher facilitated a final project meeting in October 2011 where all project partner organisations and a local council representative met to discuss "stewardship" of the stories and agree on a protocol for seeking permission to reuse the stories for any new purpose. The resulting protocol involved approaching all four original partner organisations with a proposal to reuse the stories. Where possible, the relevant partner organisation would then approach the storyteller directly to seek their permission to reuse the stories for a new purpose that wasn't originally intended in the project ethics and consent process. While this additional process of seeking consent for reuse *wasn't a requirement* of the original ethics approval and consent process (i.e. the project partners could reuse the images in related forums and purposes), the project partners agreed that it was a mark of respect for the storytellers to seek their permission to reuse stories wherever possible. This agreement did not, in hindsight, cover the hard copies of the photos and stories that were used in the public exhibition. It also required partner organisations to retain and voluntarily act upon institutional memory and agreed processes around the digital copies of the stories. Hard copies of the story photos were all handed to the District Health Coalition acting manager to caretake and frame, mainly due to the amount of space they would require to store safely. Partner representatives debated and discussed the pros and cons of keeping the exhibition together as a whole or splitting the printed and framed images up between them. At the end of the meeting participants resolved to try to display the full exhibition as a whole at other future events around the state and then split up the framed images for display in the town where they were created. One partner representative remarked that she thought it was only fitting that the stories would be returned to the community where they were authored. Others agreed with this statement. Each partner organisation was given a DVD copy of the stories with written instructions on how they were to be used. Thus began a period of relatively disparate and unknown mediation of the project stories as the project came to an official end and the partners continued on with their daily work.

The researcher handed over the university's DVD copy of the digital stories to a research centre administrator to store as confidential research data on a research data repository at the conclusion of the photographer's contract. The researcher included a written notification of the agreed process for reusing the stories with the DVD of files. Instructions on how to use the stories were also included on a file on the DVD titled "Read this first!" Just one week after the final meeting of project partners, the researcher received an email that was sent to all researchers in the centre asking for their feedback on the centre's new marketing materials and templates. The researcher opened the new marketing templates and found that two images included in a graphical banner were from the project stories. This was not an approved use of the story images. As caretaker of the stories, the researcher immediately advised staff within the research centre that the marketing materials should not be approved until the agreed process for seeking consent for reuse had been undertaken with the original project partners. The researcher then wrote to the project partner representatives to formally seek permission to reuse the images for this purpose in the marketing materials. Only two partner representatives replied to the email requesting permission to reuse the story images in the research centre's marketing materials due to its status as a not-for-profit institution. They both indicated that they thought it was OK to use the images in this way. As story caretaker the researcher experienced years of individual discomfort and feelings of misappropriation regarding this use of the story images. After taking a new job in a new area of the university, she resigned herself to this use of the stories as something she could not change.

In May 2013, almost exactly two years after the project exhibition was held, the researcher was contacted by the Director of her research centre at the university asking if she would be able to represent the institution at a National Reconciliation Week (see http://www.reconciliation.org.au/nrw/what-is-nrw/) event. The event involved the state health department "handing back" the project hard copy images to the Aboriginal housing organisation which was one of the original project partner organisations. The invitation to attend this event had come from the state health department to the head of school at the university. This was intriguing at the time given that the head of school had not been linked in any way to the project previously. The researcher attended the event, which was held at the district hospital in the town where the stories were created. At the event she found that only two of the original project partners – the Chair and CEO of the Aboriginal housing organisation – were present. The images of participants who had been recruited via their organisation were being returned to display in the organisation's offices. After speaking to the Chair of the housing organisation in 2016 we became aware that the photos had taken "pride of place" in the hospital for some time. This listening environment had been negotiated by the Health Coalition partner representative sometime after the project's official completion. The Chair of the housing organisation remarked that he felt the "visual aspect" of the display at the hospital was "empowering for the local community" and was a positive reminder that "a proper partnership can work". As he looked back over the photos of the 2011 exhibition launch with the researcher in 2016, the Chair said: "see, you can really see that she [the photographer] was listening [to the storytellers] and that made a difference."

The researcher, who was at the time heavily focused on processes of listening and mediation in preparation for this book, was intrigued with the political aspects of what had happened to the project stories after the official project end and – indeed – the continuing life story of the project after that time. It was highly significant for her that the photos were "returned" to an original project partner by representatives of a hospital as part of Reconciliation Week – an event heavily weighted with meaning in Australia. For the researcher, the process of "handing back" the photos was conative of the handing back of Aboriginal skeletal remains of ancestors removed from Australia by British governments and museums during colonisation. Hence, at least for the researcher, the stories had been "taken up" in a stream of longer-term meta-narrative and meta-oratory institutional processes regarding colonisation and reconciliation between British European invaders and First Nations peoples. At its extreme, one could interpret the appropriation of the stories and their benevolent return as ongoing acts of colonial violence and oppression. When she spoke to the Chair of the Aboriginal housing organisation in 2016 and shared a draft of this case study, the researcher asked "am I going overboard here?" The Chair replied that he and the CEO of the housing organisation had seen things in a possibly less politicised way at the time of the handing back and hadn't thought much of it other than "where are we going to put all these photos?!" During their conversation, though, the Chair said that he could see the researcher's point and thought that these observations should remain in the case study.

The lack of institutional memory which positioned the state health department as paternalistic "giver" reiterates familiar ways of imagining and talking about Aboriginal people in Australia. By this stage in the project's afterlife it could easily appear to newcomers that the project was an initiative of the state health department and not the result of a true partnership. In this way, the state health department had become an institutional meta-orator who reframed the project and its stories and hence their potential social and political significance and meaning in this listening environment. There was no acknowledgement of the photographer, the storytellers, or any of the project partners during the handing-over ceremony that day. There was also no indication that the stories that were being handed back to the Aboriginal housing organisation had actually been jointly created *by that organisation* years before in partnership with local storytellers and other project partners. There was no evidence that any of the original storytellers were present and no information provided regarding their consent to have their stories shared via the hospital walls as an unexpected listening environment. Hence the processes that led to this visible step in recontextualising and remediating the stories were a virtual "black box" to most if not all attendees at the event, including the researcher. It is in such elisions and reframings that forms of oppression and privilege are arguably and potentially reproduced.

A further two years after this in December 2015 the researcher's director asked her to initiate the process of seeking partner and participant consent to reprint selected images from the collection to display at a 20-year celebration of the research centre's work. The research director suggested that the centre could then frame and display the images long term at the university for all to see. The researcher initiated the agreed process and the project partners responded via email. A subsequent process was undertaken by partner representatives at the Aboriginal housing organisation to seek additional approval from the original storytellers to reproduce their stories for this purpose at the university. In undertaking this process – the most recent in the project's life story – the researcher, as one of the story caretakers, felt that some kind of justice and reconciliation had been achieved through once again making the process of mediation and consent transparent and visible as opposed to the black box of mediation that had occurred in the intervening years.

These are only the mediations that we know about. This case study is based on the artefacts and recollections offered by a very small number of the project partner representatives. It is consequently just a partial telling of the broader project life story and its ongoing mediation (see Table 2.1).

Theorising listening: Curators, hosts, caretakers, and brokers of listening

We would like to pause now in the chapter to theorise some of the practice we have described so far. As reflected in the above case study and discussion of listening occasions, all opportunities for listening to digital stories are curated or hosted to some degree. As evident in the case study above, we have come to use the terms *curator* and *host* to differentiate between listening environments that are created to facilitate listening to particular selections of stories – such as galleries or museums that display a specific "collection" of stories – and more "anonymous" and generalised hosting platforms (such as Facebook) where content is less directly influenced by third parties. Curated collections are often themed or fit within a metanarrative and may be gathered together with a particular purpose in mind. An example of a curated collection of stories is the UN4U digital photography contests held by the United Nations Development Programme in 2014. The UN4U competition organisers called for submissions of original photos via Instagram or email on the theme of

Table 2.1 Examples of online and offline listening occasions and environments described in current literature and storytelling projects

Listening environment	Online or offline access, continuity, levels of interaction	Aims	Description and applications	Examples and further reading
In-person digital storytelling and listening occasions	Typically offline May be transferred to online Limited access Non-enduring One to one One to few	Therapy Support Community building Reinforcing existing action Skill development Story development Recreation	Storytellers create their stories together and share the finished product with other storytellers and facilitators. Stories are shared in "draft" and final form with others e.g. in story circles Research projects seeking to understand the patient experience and how patients and families can support one another through digital storytelling. Support groups between patients and/or family members of patients. Classroom digital storytelling and sharing Recreational storytelling projects e.g. in aged care	Wilson et al. (2015)
Broadcast media	Offline Ephemeral Non-enduring without reproduction One to many Few to many Many to many	News Public information Awareness raising Entertainment Education Community building	Broadcast quality stories on a particular theme of interest to broadcast media audiences e.g. everyday lives of the Welsh or life of an asylum seeker in Australia	*Capture Wales*
Geographical information systems (GIS) mapped stories	Online Enduring Constant access One to many Few to many Many to many	Awareness raising Education Advocacy Emplaced storytelling	GIS mapped storytelling is used when the location of the story is significant to its content or potential use/impact. The story is presented on a map of a neighbourhood, city, region, country, or the world to show the context from which the story emerges. Often used in collaborative place-based storytelling projects.	Hiroshima Testimonies: http://hiroshima.archiving.jp/index_en.html Partition Archive of British India: http://www.1947partitionarchive.org/

Listening environment	Online or offline access, continuity, levels of interaction	Aims	Description and applications	Examples and further reading
Organisational marketing or promotion	Online Constant access Potentially enduring Few to many	Marketing Public relations Support Fundraising	Stories of service user or beneficiary experiences intended to shed a positive light on the hosting organisation Stories of how non-profit organisations have supported service users. Intended to demonstrate impact. May provide testimony/reviews to encourage new service users	Redkite cancer support non-profit: http://www.redkite.org.au/real-stories?gclid=CIOhprXolsoCFUccvAodCo0B6Q
Public exhibition (static or mobile)	Offline Digital artefacts may be offered online Limited access (physical presence required) Non-enduring One to few One to many Few to few Few to many	Personal expression Self-representation Awareness raising Education Advocacy Network and community building	Digital stories are displayed in a public setting for listening Mobile exhibitions of digital stories e.g. a van, portable display, or rickshaw Relocatable exhibition kiosks e.g. touchscreen units in remote locations that have unreliable Internet access Art gallery, museum, or other organisation's exhibition of digital stories in an established public or private building	eTuktuk initiative Sri Lanka: http://www.etuktuk.net/ (see also Tacchi & Grubb, 2007; Tacchi, Watkins, & Keerthirathne, 2009) Storybank India: http://www.cs.swan.ac.uk/tellingstorybank/index.php Home to Home exhibition – young Australians with disability living in nursing homes: http://www.eventfinda.com.au/2015/home-to-home-digital-story-exhibition/geelong
Digital archive – public or restricted access	Typically online Constant access, may be restricted to certain users Enduring Many to many	Preservation Rejuvenation Transmission Recording testimony Advocacy Human rights	Collections of stories that are deliberately created and protected to preserve knowledge and experience of the storytellers Endangered language and culture storytelling and preservation Survivor testimony Healing and reconciliation projects Archives of websites that have ceased to be publicly available	Stolen Generations testimonies Australia: http://stolengenerationstestimonies.com/index.php/about_stolen_generations.html Digital Archive of Cambodian Holocaust Survivors: http://www.cybercambodia.com/dachs/stories.html British Library archive of oral history websites: http://www.webarchive.org.uk/ukwa/collection/65208410/page/1

Listening environment	Online or offline access, continuity, levels of interaction	Aims	Description and applications	Examples and further reading
Public open access, hosted, curated	Online Constant access Potentially enduring Many to many	Self-representation Awareness raising Education Advocacy Research Public relations Marketing	Open calls for stories on a particular theme e.g. human rights, gender inequality, the environment, ageing, or disability used for advocacy, research, or policymaking purposes Stories intended to provide support to others who are experiencing similar life events to the storyteller e.g. Beyond Blue Australia's Personal Stories collection https://www.beyondblue.org.au/connect-with-others/personal-stories Story collections used for research, training, or professional development Websites and social media versions of broadcast media content available on demand	Patient Voices: http://www.patientvoices.org.uk/stories.htm Colorectal Cancer Digital Story-telling Project (via YouTube): https://www.youtube.com/playlist?list=PL331E196C4C64383D The HUB human rights participatory media site: http://hub.witness.org/en/AboutHub
Public open access, hosted, self-curated	Online Constant access Potentially enduring Many to many	Personal expression Self-representation Entertainment Self-education Education Public relations Marketing	Personal profiles and blogs Personal websites on open access public platforms such as Google sites	Brain Injury Community: From Survivors to Thrivers, Ken Aiken blog: https://braininjurycommunity.wordpress.com/ My wife's fight with breast cancer: http://mywifesfightwithbreastcancer.com/blog/ YouTube, Facebook, Blogspot, Instagram, Google sites

gender inequality. Winners of UN4U photography competitions are often used as advocates and champions for social change via blogs and social media profiles. Another interesting example of curation of a group of stories might be Brenda Bruggeman's role in pulling together and introducing digital stories from the US Digital Archive of Literacy Narratives (DALN) around Deaf identity and literacy into an "exhibition" of stories within the collection (Comer & Harker, 2015). In such cases, particularly where autobiographical texts are not generated within workshop settings but are sent in by storytellers, the role of curator as opposed to facilitator or host of stories is particularly clear.

In contrast to curators, hosts can simply provide an environment for listening without any particular knowledge of or control over story content. Hosts that don't employ a curatorial role are typically more concerned with creating spaces and environments and providing an environment for "guests" to attend those spaces to share or listen to stories, in the same way one might host a dinner party by providing the space and basic resources needed to come and have a good time. An example of a hosted but not necessarily curated listening environment might include YouTube, Vimeo, Instagram, or Google sites. As with all media the hosting environment will have some influence on which kinds of content can be shared and how content is presented, e.g. within a broader frame of a YouTube profile/website.

We have mapped out in the case study above the role of story caretaker. This role can be distinct from – but also potentially overlapping with – both the curating and hosting roles. Caretaking involves monitoring the ethical use and reuse of mediated stories that have been moved from the original story-teller. Our conversations with practitioners suggest that in building in ethical practices of seeking consent, generating stories, and negotiating the conditions under which those stories might be listened to, storytelling facilitators often take on roles as story caretakers, at least in the early phases of a storytelling project (e.g. Gubrium et al., 2014). Where story collection has been built into the roles and routines of large institutions, as we will see when discussing the roles of patient experience managers in the Welsh NHS in Chapter four, those caretaking roles may be ongoing, if under-recognised and under-resourced. Others we have spoken to underline the limits of their capacity to care for stories, especially those emerging in international contexts, and stress the role of partner or commissioning organisations in this ongoing role. In the case study above, the photographer, who was the facilitator of the photovoice activities, also acted as curator, and for a time, caretaker of the stories. The researcher then took over the caretaking role after the photographer's contract ended.

In the case of commercially hosted environments for storytelling and listening such as personal websites, social media profiles, and blogs there is often an interesting mixture of the roles of host, curator, and caretaker. The storyteller/ host of personal sites also plays a meta-oratory role as curator of his or her own collection of story artefacts. Depending on their intentions, storytellers can play a more or less pronounced "curating" role in the presentation of their autobiographical materials. A user who hosts a website to promote awareness of acquired brain injury and support fellow brain injury survivors for example may be more interested in actively *hosting* a site for others – i.e. for listeners – than deliberately *curating* a particular collection of stories. The standard personal Facebook site is an example where users oscillate along a continuum of more and less conscious curatorship of their own self-representation. Users draw on their self-authored posts, images, videos, and re-presentation of material authored by other people to create and curate a representation of themselves over time.

Tanja Dreher in her recent work suggests that in order to generate a wider range of listeners, digital stories also need support from *brokers*. Dreher (2012) sees a broker as an agent with some institutional power, for instance, members of funding bodies or policymakers within government departments that may have commissioned a particular set of digital stories, who can create links to new hosts – such as broadcasters – and their viewers and listeners. Higher education teachers and professional educators using collections of stories in classrooms, particularly those publicising and promoting online archives like the US Digital Archive of Literacy Narratives (DALN) as well as using them in their own practice, could be seen as acting as brokers (Comer & Harker, 2015). Equally, researchers, especially action researchers, could be considered brokers: for example, Locock and her colleagues (Locock et al., 2014) in their work using narratives from *HealthTalkOnline* as part of an experience-based co-design project in which staff and patients worked together on redesigning systems and processes, using discussions catalysed by listening to digital stories.

All four of these meta-oratory roles can influence the presentation context and meta-narratives that surround digital stories. People and organisations who inhabit these roles as meta-orators contribute a layer of contextual meaning to any presentation of digital stories and consequently, these roles are politically and ethically significant. Nancy Thumim (2009) for example draws attention to the ways that institutional collections of stories such as the Museum of London's *London's Voices* and BBC Wales' *Capture Wales* mediate and "curate" participant stories in several important ways. She notes in particular the somewhat illusionary nature of the stories representing "everyday" and "ordinary" people's voices in what is often a relatively highly produced outcome of several waves of institutional mediation. Here the "ordinary" individual's voice becomes intermingled with institutional voices that call upon various professional, disciplinary, and personal discourses of decision makers and technicians alike. Thumim (2009) also draws our attention to the processes of archiving and labelling through metadata that shape the rhetorical and moral [re]delivery, historicising, and future potential [re]listenings of stories that have already been "used", "seen", or "heard" through some form of public exhibition or broadcast – a process we will explore in more detail in the second half of this chapter.

If digital storytelling projects aim towards democratisation and social justice, all of these meta-oratory roles are implicated in the success or otherwise of such aspirations. As the above case study indicates, a caretaking role can honour agreements with original storytellers regarding reuse and controlling the remediation and recontextualisation of stories in a way that actually inhibits their use for policymaking or social justice purposes. In this way mediated stories can become *tethered* to the original storyteller in both time and space in a way that limits the reach of their potential impact in social contexts outside of the storytellers' and project partners' immediate political, cultural, and social spheres of influence, experience, or imagination. This ethical tethering of stories was evident in the case study to the degree that the story caretakers attempted to maintain a constant consent process from original storytellers in any reuse of their stories in new listening environments, where understandings of what could be seen and where had not previously been negotiated.

None of the case study project's stories were ever made available in an online form of any kind. Their recontextualisation in a digital form was limited to DVD format and secure institutional networks. In one case the protocols for sharing the stories and the fact that they were not available publicly online may have resulted in a limiting of local council members' access to the stories for listening which, ironically, may have resulted in the limiting of their potential to effect social change for social justice. This is not to say that a process could not have been pursued in order to grant special permission for the council members to listen to the stories via a new hosting relationship and listening environment such as council meetings. In this particular case study (as we expect in many others as well) the project had ended and the process of establishing new consent processes for this avenue of listening was not pursued. The prospect of stories being used for purposes or listened to by audiences their tellers would not be happy with is the key ethical threat articulated in most accounts of digital storytelling (Gubrium et al., 2014; Hardy & Sumner, 2014; Vivienne & Burgess, 2012). However, the tale of the case study project stories, and many of the conversations we have had with practitioners, suggest quite a different set of potential problems. These challenges point to the importance of the roles of caretakers and hosts, as well as facilitators, in creating ethical routes towards wider groups of listeners.

The challenges of institutional meta-oration

The first case study above exemplifies the complexity and messiness of using digital stories – or any other form of human stories about personal experience – for "applied" political purposes. In her work on the *Capture Wales* project, Thumim (2009, p. 617) concluded that the BBC and Museum of London's "institutional power is not fundamentally altered" by their privileging of personal stories as part of their institutional collections and broadcasting. Thumim's work draws us to consider once again the realities of the so-called "democratising" functions of digital storytelling when applied to the relationship of storytellers and institutional curators. The fact that the case study stories were removed and then repatriated to the Aboriginal Housing agency that originally partnered in the storytelling project was an indication that existing power relations and social orders were not arguably durably challenged but rather were reproduced in the context of the case study's extended project life (i.e. after the time of the planned and negotiated public exhibition of the stories). It appears that institutions such as museums, broadcasters, and by extension governments can gather and present first-person accounts with little disruption to their commonplace power and privilege as a *meta-orator* in and of public life. As Nick Couldry (2012) emphasised, media can work to disrupt or reproduce the social order. Digital storytelling artefacts and the listening environments via which we access them are no exceptions to this statement.

The outcomes of institutions taking on meta-oratory roles need to be thoroughly considered. For example, we interviewed staff involved in a digital storytelling project run by a local city council with local refugees and asylum seekers. In this project, the roles of institutions as meta-orators appeared to be an accepted part of mediation processes. It was a condition or outcome of grant monies for the project that the funding and partner institutions would take on some form of "ownership" of personal story artefacts that arise from digital storytelling. Here the copyright over a digital story can vary from who is the story maker or author. Institutional ownership of story artefacts can both produce and inhibit listening. In this context, storytellers were initially told that their stories would be shared via the local council's website to promote awareness of asylum-seeker and refugee experiences and needs in the broader community. In the end the stories were not shared on any public website due to an assessment that the digital stories were "poor quality". It was a marketing department decision ultimately whether or not these stories would be shared on the council website. At the time of preparing this book the stories were stored digitally on a secure server at the local council's library but were not offered online or publicly in any ongoing fashion. When we asked the project manager if another partner organisation such as a non-profit organisation might be willing to host the stories on their website, the project manager raised the issue of copyright and ownership of the stories. She commented: "Whose stories are they really? Are they Council's? If so is there any issue with another organisation sharing them?"

As we will explore elsewhere in the book, the conflation of individual storytellers' voice with institutional voices is most apparent in listening environments that are hosted or curated by professional media and public relations representatives. Here the curatorial role can take on a particular focus and intention in making the institution look good – that is, socially responsible, ethical, engaged – to outside audiences via its selection and display of citizen-authored digital stories. Even as it uses the language of ethical engagement, this curatorial intentionality and selectivity can depart significantly from other types of curatorship that are focused on social justice, health, or well-being content and themes.

The threats of such institutional re-curating are acknowledged by Amy Hill from Silence Speaks. She notes: "We definitely have seen with some of our partners in the global public health context that there's a really big disconnect between programmatic people that we might have worked with on a project, and marketing and communication people who view the stories as tools for marketing and communications" (personal communication). Moving beyond the role of facilitator into the role of caretaker, Hill shared with us strategies for attempting to pre-empt inappropriate public relations-oriented uses of sensitive stories. She describes, for instance, an orientation activity developed for all members of a partner organisation, including those in marketing and communications positions, stressing how to contextualise and present stories, followed by a form asking all staff to agree to particular ethical protocols in their use of stories. As Hill commented on the limits of her ability to act as caretaker for stories developed in international settings: "I can't actually police and say they're actually doing that but those are the kinds of things that I feel I need to do for my own peace of mind – I can only hope these tools and recommendations are used by the organizations I work with" (personal communication). As we will observe in Chapter four, the lines between promoting participation and promoting the appearance of participation can sometimes be very blurred.

Digital listening infrastructures

Many organisations that seek to draw on digital stories for social justice ends aim to cultivate an ongoing relationship with storytellers, viewing them as partners, members, co-researchers, or co-creators within ongoing organisations and campaigns. While such ongoing relationships are widely perceived as an ideal towards which organisations using digital stories aim, the reality of digital storytelling projects has not always matched this ideal. Indeed, the use of recorded stories rather than live self-advocacy or storytelling is often a strategy to cope with situations where storytellers are not able to have an ongoing presence – for example, where storytellers have progressive medical conditions that make them less and less able to speak for themselves – or when large numbers of stories from diverse experiences and locations are desired for, for example, evidence-informed national policymaking (see also Matthews & Sunderland, 2013). Online archives of multimedia autobiographical stories are one solution to these problems.

In this section of the chapter we will discuss some of the more important archives that focus on stories of health, well-being, and disability – particularly *HealthTalkOnline* and *Patient Voices* – and some larger archives – for example those at the *StoryCenter* and *Storycorps* – that include a body of narratives on this thematising health, well-being, and disability. We ask what kinds of listening environments are created by the architectures of these digital platforms. We also analyse some of the ways that digital listening infrastructures might be organised, and some of the implications of these listening environments.

The following case studies were prepared using documentary and multimedia evidence available in the public sphere, in addition to documents provided by Pip Hardy from Patient Voices and Amy Hill from Silence Speaks. They were also supplemented by in-depth interviews conducted between 2014 and 2016. Formal interviews were conducted under an approved ethics protocol via Macquarie University. Stakeholders in this case study have only been identified based on their express request to be so.

As noted at the beginning of the chapter, "specific" digital storytelling projects, and sometimes broader photovoice, place-based storytelling, and other multimedia life narrative projects are often part-funded by institutions – broadcasters, museums or libraries, government departments, local councils, universities, or non-government organisations – institutions which may favour a non-commercial, bespoke platform for stories. Despite the costs of establishing and maintaining them, such bespoke digital sites appear to have a number of advantages. Often storytelling projects seek to establish and maintain an ongoing relationship with their storytellers for a number of reasons: to ensure a thorough consent process for circulation of the stories (Sonke Gender Justice, n.d.); to encourage storytellers to be empowered to produce further narratives (Sunderland, Chenoweth, Matthews & Ellem, 2015); or to encourage a sense of community among storytellers and between storytellers and their listeners (Vivienne & Burgess, 2012). Some bespoke platforms, like their "native" commercial counterparts, also offer the facility for storytellers to upload multimedia narratives themselves (Sunderland et al., 2015; Vivienne & Burgess, 2012). The 1000 Voices site and The Rainbow Family Tree site are both examples of this kind of architecture. These sites, developed specifically to host collections of stories, are not shaped by the constraints and affordances – and commercial considerations – of existing host platforms like YouTube or Vimeo (see for example, Fuchs, 2014; Van Dijck, 2013). There is potential to shape the listening and viewing experience on these bespoke platforms in ways that might reflect the ethical and social justice commitments of those running storytelling projects. However, simply deciding not to use these commercial host platforms, with their well-known ethical challenges around unpaid labour and data mining, does not mean that bespoke sites sidestep the shaping processes of mediatisation.

While an ongoing online presence might seem to offer digital alternatives to the roles of caretaker or broker, in fact a web presence for a collection of stories requires ongoing caretaking (Sunderland et al., 2015). At the most practical level, this caretaking involves maintenance, management, and updating of the site. As we have argued elsewhere (Sunderland et al., 2015), encouraging and facilitating participation continues to have a significant role even for sites devised to allow participants to upload stories themselves. This is particularly the case for storytellers who might not be easily able to access digital technologies or have the particular digital literacies or physical and intellectual capacity required to manage autonomous uploading of materials. More broadly, attempts to manage the interface between a bespoke site with its often carefully negotiated ethical protocols for use of materials and the wider terrain of the Internet beyond with its shared cultural practices around copying, commenting, rating, parodies, and mash-ups have often involved a kind of ethical caretaking.

Some sites that have very clear "owners" – for instance, Patient Voices, which has since the early 2000s been run as a social enterprise by Pip Hardy and Tony Sumner, or the site of StoryCenter – have professionals who undertake professionalised digital storytelling caretaking, brokering, hosting, and curatorship roles. Both these sites are very visibly curated by their founders and long-term caretakers, whose ongoing labour to maintain the site and ensure ongoing consent from storytellers to have their narratives hosted there are significant if often understated in popular understandings of the status of collections of online material.

In our own experiences with digital storytelling projects and our surveying of the literature, the role of broker is often significant for online collections of stories, as new listeners are sought for the stories and new uses are made of existing resources. An important example would be the research on service improvement produced by Locock and colleagues from the British online site *HealthTalkOnline*. While *HealthTalkOnline*, drawn from an ongoing collection of narratives for health research, is framed primarily as a resource for patient and public information, it has also come to be used as a resource for professional education and service improvement. While there are traces of such uses in the welcome videos on the site, the diversity of applications of stories across patient and professional uses is more visible in research published by Locock and colleagues. These research projects have drawn from the collection of video narratives as part of service improvement projects, brokering and remediatising for new listeners and new uses (Locock et al., 2014). Teachers and trainers can also serve as both brokers and curators of selections of digital stories. Tony Sumner from Pilgrim Projects notes, for instance, that a "vast majority of hits on the website don't go down the little walk through web pages to find a story that's of interest. The vast majority go straight to a particular story, because someone has already put that link into a learning program" (personal communication).

Affordances of bespoke infrastructures for health-related narratives

Lawrence Lessig, in his early and influential corrective to libertarian accounts of new media, with their simplistic binaries of freedom and constraint, deploys the word "regulation" to discuss online architectures. Just as, often without drawing attention to the constraints it imposes, architecture shapes how we can move and interact in "real space" as Lessig calls it, "the software and hardware that make cyberspace what it is constitute a set of constraints on how you can behave" (Lessig, 1999, p. 89). Rather than seeing regulation simply as the rules imposed by government, Lessig's much broader account includes the way markets, social norms, and architectures, as well as legal frameworks, shape behaviour. As Shilton (2015) argues in more recent work, exploring the ways in which ethics might be embedded in software engineering, "values are … concretized in design choices and system rules" (p. 2). As she points out, the affordances of software systems may privilege some users while marginalising others (Shilton, 2015, p. 5). While we recognise that the ways in which software platforms are used are diverse and unpredictable (see Van Dijck, 2013, p. 33), in this section we want to think through the possible outcomes of the affordances of platforms built to host digital stories.

Jean Burgess and Joshua Green in their book on YouTube (Burgess & Green, 2009) turn towards content in their analysis, as a corrective to what they see as an excessive focus on architectures on the one hand and rich ethnographic accounts of small numbers of participants on the other. However, as we have argued throughout this book, the digital storytelling literature has focused primarily on process and on small-scale, if rich, accounts of the content of particular stories. Consequently we focus here on the navigation and metaoration functions of hosting platforms rather than the much more widely discussed content of digital storytelling collections.

Our aim is not to set up a tick list of "right" and "wrong" ways to host digital stories. As we've argued throughout this book, while we celebrate and share the social justice commitments of those commissioning and facilitating digital storytelling programs, the language of "ought" and "should" has sometimes been a straitjacket for thinking about how stories have been and can be used. Rather we want to explore some of the possible consequences, both fruitful and challenging, of particular decisions about the way that bespoke platforms for hosting stories might present, by considering some quite different approaches to the core features of particular sites. In making this argument we draw on Van Dijck's (2013) insight that "different sites' architectures cultivate different styles of connectedness, self-presentation and taste performance" (p. 34).

Online repositories of digital stories have proliferated in recent years. As we have argued in earlier work, the use of databases is a logical consequence of the citizen-to-citizen mode of dissemination imagined by many emphasising the value of digital storytelling for social change (Matthews & Sunderland, 2013). This is particularly the case where peer information sharing is the primary outcome imagined for digital storytelling, as in the case of the long-standing and substantial *HealthTalkOnline* site (previously known as DipEx). However, even in the limited instances where digital stories are used in more structured contexts for education, policy development, or service improvement, databases of stories are often developed as resources to enable that outcome. For instance, the Telling Stories website, hosted by the UK NHS's National Genetics and Genomics Education Centre, hosts life experience narratives in various forms by people who have been diagnosed as having a genetic condition. It has been primarily developed as a teaching resource in the undergraduate education of nurses, midwives, and doctors. Nonetheless both the stories and teaching material associated with them are hosted online as part of a database. While the embedding of these stories in the curriculum structures the way that learners will listen to them and think through them, the architecture, notably the way it facilitates what Couldry has described as the most fundamental digital media practice – searching (Couldry, 2012, p. 45; see also Simonsen,

2011) – will also play a role in structuring the listening experience of those encountering the database.

We now explore some key features of a number of bespoke publicly accessible databases of multimodal life experience narratives which incorporate information about health, well-being, or disability. We will focus on *Telling Stories, HealthTalkOnline, Patient Voices* (all based in the UK), and *1000 Voices* (based in Australia). While our emphasis is on collections of life experience narratives that foreground questions of health, we will also include some discussion of wider collections of stories – *StoryCorps, Storycenter,* and the *Digital Archive of Literacy Narratives* (DALN) (each based in the US) – which include a number of stories thematising health.

Case study: How digital infrastructures shape listening

The title and the theme of a repository play a potentially important part in the meta-oratory of a collection of stories. The "look" of the site and its name serve in framing the listening environment for individual stories. Krista Bryson (2012) for example, has argued that the titling of the large collection of narratives around reading, writing, and multimedia literacies – the *Digital Archive of Literacy Narratives* (DALN) – as well as the key images used to illustrate the notion of literacy, narrows the range of interpretations of the archives in ways that support a rather conservative understanding of literacy, despite the more open-ended views of the project initiators and steering group (p. 259). It is worth considering whether the foregrounding of health, disability, or patient-hood in the title or framing of projects like *Patient Voices* or *HealthTalkOnline* frames diverse and meaning-rich narratives. Well aware of the problems of the language of medicalisation, Pip Hardy and Tony Sumner of Pilgrim Projects express some frustration about most people's take on the title of their database of "classic" digital stories about health and well-being. Tony comments, "Patient Voices was never really about patients. It was about the voices that were waiting patiently to be heard, or to be listened to" (personal communication). From the perspective of activists who use the social model of disability as a key tool, or indeed from a minority rights perspective on disability, navigation terms like Deaf or disability might be seen as less problematic than more directly biomedical terms.

In methodological debates over archiving, analysing, and deploying large numbers of life story narratives a key issue is the integrity of individual stories. Many writers using life stories for research and many practitioners involved in collecting digital stories and other forms of mediated life story, remain concerned about preserving, and the dangers of fragmenting or reframing, the storyteller's account. Pip Hardy summarises this position in her account of the views of the very first storytellers for Patient Voices, whose ideas deeply shaped the way stories came to be collected and used. These storytellers put the case that, "Once we're happy with our story, we don't want some researcher to dismember it, and just take the bits they like" (personal communication).

Part of the purpose of collecting multimodal stories is to preserve the richness of the narrative, voice, and preferred mode of communication of the story's author. Consequently, academic work drawing on life narrative, even research that draws on large numbers of life stories or life histories, has tended to privilege the case study because of the way case studies preserve the integrity and framing of the story. This emphasis on the case study and reluctance to pull apart stories into their constituent fragments or themes for the purpose of analysis, we have argued in previous work, has been one key reason for the difficulty of using collections of life story narratives for research and policymaking (Matthews & Sunderland, 2013). As John Hartley (2007) has suggested, these issues have given digital storytelling a problem with scalability. These same debates emerge in examining the architectures of the online databases of stories. We would suggest there is an inherent tension between the usability of large collections of stories and the preservation of their integrity.

Various collections of health service user life narratives have tackled this problem differently. On one end of the spectrum, the stories of *HealthTalkOnline* – which largely constitute videoed interviews – are segmented, with each page containing a series of extracts, sometimes from the same person or recording occasions, sometimes from a diversity of different perspectives. These segments are woven together with a clear, authoritative written text with no obvious personal voice or author. The voice of expertise in *HealthTalkOnline* visibly sutures together these thematised chunks of various video narratives. While the scale of the *HealthTalkOnline* site is huge, the ways in which resources are presented make this site feel more curated than hosted.

Telling Stories, a site bringing together narratives around genetics for audiences of nurses, doctors, and medical educators, as well as for patients, incorporates stories that are generally kept as a whole, rather than being sliced and diced. However, because the aim of the site is to provide learning resources for both self-motivated learners and nurse educators, it frames the stories it includes much more directly in terms of learning outcomes and issues to reflect on. The guiding voice of the educator is there in the "Toolkit" box which flags up points for reflection, activities, and identifies key quotations. A separate section of each page links the story to nursing, midwifery, medical student, and general practitioner competencies.

Unsurprisingly, sites like *1000 Voices* and *Patient Stories* choose not to fragment the narratives they host. As we noted earlier, one of the key underpinning philosophies of the digital storytelling movement has been the notion that editing is the terrain of the storyteller and that mediators and gatekeepers should be minimised. These sites, then, include very little in the way of the narrative voice of an expert meta-orator. Unlike *Telling Stories* or *HealthTalkOnline*, stories are not woven together or explained through an overarching medical or pedagogical frame. Stories appear with little in the way of introduction or contextualisation. In some senses, the stories and the storytellers here speak for themselves. However, even sites like these that actively work to displace expert voices are embedded within the context of the meta-oratory of the site itself. The site's organisation and its navigation – features like headings, word-clouds, tags, and menus – serve as meta-orators.

Theorising listening: directing listening through infrastructure navigation and design

Navigation and the focusing illusion

G. Thomas Couser, one of the most prominent writers on memoir, specifically autobiographical work by people with illness or disability (Couser, 1997, 2004, 2012), has recently argued for the value of life story in the health care sector. He begins by noting the disparity between the assessments of their own quality of life of people with disability and the assessments made of such people's quality of life by the general public, including health care workers (see also Sunderland et al., 2009). Couser (2014) describes this as "a hidden *impairment:* a massive collective mindblindness in nondisabled people, especially health-care professionals, who are unable to imagine what disabled people are thinking and feeling" (p. 2). Drawing on the work of Amundson and the concept of hedonics, he argues that self-representations have the potential to mitigate against this mind blindness.

Hedonics involves the study of pleasure and happiness. Ron Amundson (2010) notes that the most powerful impact on assessments of quality of life is "the focussing illusion" (p. 384). When people are encouraged to focus on a particular aspect of their lives which has significance for their assessment of their quality of life (for instance, whether they have been dating recently or not), their subsequent overall assessment of quality of life is impacted. Two people who have similar success in dating, for example, will offer very different assessments of their quality of life depending on whether they have been asked to ruminate on their dating experiences first. Drawing on this work, Couser (2014) argues that life experience accounts that are holistic, like the memoir of a person with an impairment, may offer material to fuel a very different assessment of the quality of life of people with disability by people who, due to limited personal experience, otherwise might focus on the impairments of the person with disability (p. 4).

This work offers some insights into the challenges of setting up a database of life experience stories by people with disability or health conditions. The ways in which the material is organised and tagged shape its searchability and usability. However, the ways in which stories are categorised and labelled also have the potential to shape the ways in which the life stories within the database are listened to. If the architecture and tagging of stories emphasise impairment, the focusing illusion is likely to be brought into play. Linzi Juliano and Ramesh Srinivasan have argued, for instance, that crowd-sourced tags tend to constrain and fix the divergent meanings of online objects (Juliano & Srinivasan, 2012, p. 616). This is a very different understanding of crowd-sourced tagging from more utopian accounts that emphasised the value of a wider, non-professionalised public playing a role in classifying and ordering (e.g. McKee, 2011).

An obvious difference between the life experience databases discussed here is evident in the role of medical language in categorising and tagging stories. *HealthTalkOnline*, with its primary focus on peer education and dissemination of patient information, uses diagnostic labels most extensively on their website. Their "categories" include some non-medical categories such as "men's health", "women's health", and "improving health care". However, even where their alphabetised list includes socio-cultural experiences rather than biomedical categories – items such as "birth after Caesarean", "bereavement and grieving", or "young people" – a majority of sub-categories under these labels relate to medical conditions such as "arthritis" and "epilepsy".

The disability movement has extensively critiqued medicalisation as a way of accounting for the difficulties and marginalisation experienced by disabled people, and the social model of disability has emphasised instead the social, economic, and political obstacles that disabled people with impairments experience. While *HealthTalkOnline* is organised largely around medical conditions, within the section of the website focusing on a particular position, there is a broader focus not simply on medical issues, such as experiences of symptoms, treatments, or drugs, but also on wider social or service provision, considerations that might be viewed as part of the disabling social context which makes embodied differences socially meaningful. For example, the section of *HealthTalkOnline* headed "epilepsy" includes a section on schooling and studying that incorporates a number of testimonies on experiences of bullying, while another section on transport considers the difficulties people with epilepsy may have in employment and everyday life because of the cost of public transport and the need for a car to get around many areas. Equally, the section of *HealthTalkOnline* which is organised around the profiles of individual interviewees offers a more holistic picture of the person, their social situation, and allows listeners to watch several clips from the interview that they have given at a sitting.

The *NHS Your Choices* website, which includes a range of short videos in various formats, many of which focus on an individual's narrative of their own life experience, takes a similar approach to navigation. "Sign language" for instance is a category, within which video materials using British Sign Language are included on a range of topics, reflecting at least in part a linguistic or non-biomedical view of Deafness. Social and cultural categories such as "carers" are included, but so too are medical categories like "cancer". The site titles its videos in a similar "mixed" way, using particular conditions, but also flagging up the person's name – for instance "Downs' Syndrome: Emily's Story", "Measles: Rachel's Story", or "You Only Die Once: Kate Granger's Story".

There are clearly practical advantages for public access and navigation of these sites in using biomedical terms as part of their architecture and tagging.

Indeed, for people recently diagnosed with illnesses or conditions or their families searching for first-hand experience of these illnesses, diagnostic or biomedical categories are undoubtedly a first point of call. Equally for nurses and doctors using the *Telling Stories* site to educate themselves about the human, experiential impact of genetic conditions, biomedical categories are a vital starting point. However, we can offer an example of the potential hazards of the focusing effect of navigation structures within bespoke sites from our own experience behind the scenes with the development of the *1000 Voices* site, hosted by Griffith University in Australia. One of the early and powerful contributions to the site was Phil Deschamp's (2009) written narrative "Wild Animals in Skips", accompanied by some extraordinarily beautiful photographic abstracts. Deschamp's narrative is framed in terms of the challenges of finding new, non-clichéd photographic subject matter, and artistic traditions of abstract expressionism and the Fauves. Only around halfway through his narrative does he share the particular logistical challenges of capturing in-focus close-ups of the corroded sides of waste skips posed by his physical position as a user of an electric wheelchair. His meditation on artistic value concludes as he reflects in his final paragraph: "people who start off enjoying the images can be disconcerted if I confess that I took them from the side of a dumpster". In an early iteration of the navigation and tagging structure for *1000 Voices* before it was redeveloped, this careful sequence of disclosures and framings came to be headed with tags that highlighted, before the reader had completed the narrative, that Phil was a wheelchair user. Rather than framing the narrative, as the title did, around artistic traditions, aesthetic innovation, and the repurposing of the devalued, these tags framed the narrative explicitly around disability. This reframing happened despite 1000 Voices' commitment to the voice of the storytellers and consistent work to honour the narratives and modes in which storytellers chose to speak. This example points towards something that a number of hosts of digital storytelling collections told us – that often decisions about the navigation, tagging, and categorisation of sites were less a result of active decision making than a serendipitous outcome of limited time and resources and a lack of obvious alternatives.

Other bespoke platforms take a very different approach to the top-down navigation. *Patient Voices*, for example, prioritises the individual authors in the titling of the story, and organises stories around the funded project of which they were a part. In some cases a project focuses on a particular illness or segment of the health field, for instance, the *Dangling Stories* site with people with dementia recorded in conjunction with the University of Abertay Dundee, or the stories from people who have used mental health services from the Manchester Mental Health and Social Care Trust. Some collections of stories might have titles that flag up both a disability and another part of identity: "Having a stroke: being a parent" for instance. However, the stories themselves are not normally entitled in a way that flags up medical diagnoses.

Patient Voices currently uses word clouds drawn from the text of the story as an approach foregrounding the storyteller's own words rather than using terms drawn from expert vocabularies. Word clouds might be viewed as a kind of folksonomy since they are generated from user input, although they don't function as a navigation device on this site the way tag folksonomies on sites like YouTube do. *1000 Voices* uses a word-cloud approach as a key to its "explore" function. These terms include both diagnostic terminology (e.g. palsy) and reference to enabling technologies (i.e. wheelchairs).

Navigating intimate publics

Perhaps unsurprisingly, since they share the commitments of *Patient Voices* and *1000 Voices* to the pre-eminence and integrity of the storyteller's account, the approaches to navigation taken by StoryCenter, associated with the CDS, and the large oral history project *Storycorps* are closer to those of *Patient Voices* than *HealthTalkOnline*. Stories are grouped thematically, and with storytellers' title and a key image as the visual and linguistic links. Themes include "health", "family", "relationships", or "struggle", *Storycorps* does have some collections around collective identities – notably veterans, Latino, and LGBTQI stories. *Storycorps* has a collection "Commemoration" which focuses on people with memory loss talking to friends and family. While these stories are thematised in a way that reflects the medical conditions experienced by storytellers, their title reflects the process of collecting and celebrating memories, rather than explicitly referencing a biomedical condition.

Given the frequency with which stories in both sites foreground the experience of various health conditions and impairments, we read the decision not to build biomedical conditions into the navigation of the site as a deliberate decision perhaps in response to the widely heard critiques of such labels from the disability movement over the past fifty years. Rather, the themes chosen for organising stories on these sites recall the account of the kind of public sphere that Anna Poletti identifies in "specific" digital storytelling. Poletti notes that:

> The digital storytelling movement is clear in its desire to make a con-tribution to the public sphere, and what marks that contribution as an attempt to create an intimate public is its insistence on the pre-existence of 'story' and the universality of themes such as 'life, loss, belonging, hope for the future, friendship and love' (Burgess 2006, 212).
>
> (Poletti, 2011, pp. 80–81)

While Poletti identifies these ideas – the shared human experience of story and storytelling and shared, universal thematics around the lifecycle – in the rationales for digital storytelling and in the process of constructing stories, we would argue they are also evident in the bespoke listening environments created to frame these stories.

Poletti draws on the work of Lauren Berlant, and particularly her notion of the intimate public, to attempt to make sense of the consequences of this universalising ethos in the digital storytelling movement. "What makes a public sphere intimate is an expectation that the consumers of its particular stuff already share a worldview and emotional knowledge that they have derived from a broadly common historical experience" (cited by Poletti, 2011, p. 81).

As Poletti points out, the digital storytelling "movement" is deeply invested in this notion of intimate publics – a borrowing, perhaps from progressive movements like second wave feminism with their emphasis on the personal as political. But what are the consequences of organising an archive of stories around the "universal" affective experiences Berlant and Poletti see as constituting intimate publics?

Berlant's view of the political consequences of intimate publics is a grim one:

> when sentimentality meets politics personal stories tell of structural effects, but in doing so they risk thwarting the very attempt to perform rhetorically a scene of pain that must be soothed politically. Because the ideology of true feeling cannot admit the non-universality of pain, its cases of vulnerability and suffering can become all jumbled together into a scene of the generally human, and the ethical imperative toward social transformation is replaced by a passive and vaguely civic-minded ideal of compassion. The political as a place of acts oriented towards publicness becomes replaced by a world of private thoughts, leanings, and gestures projected out as an intimate public of private individuals inhabiting their own affective changes. Suffering, in this personal/public context, becomes answered by sacrifice and survival, which is, then, recoded as the achievement of justice or liberty.
>
> (Berlant cited in Poletti, 2011, p. 80)

This account of emotional connection as quite different from political action runs very much counter to the emphasis within the digital storytelling movement on the way powerful stories can motivate change (see also Yea, 2015). While we maintain a sense of scepticism that the processes and relationships embedded in dialogic personal storytelling necessarily flow though to changes in social relationships and structures, we would suggest the roles of host, curator, caretaker, and broker can go some way towards addressing Berlant's concern that a focus on shared emotion may not address the structures that underpin inequality.

Berlant suggests that one of the problems of "intimate publics" like the ones we suggest are created by the humanist meta-oratory embedded in the search terms of these listening infrastructures, is that they often separate out the emotional story and its individual teller from the structures and institutions that created the injustice about which the storyteller might be speaking. An emotional connection with the narrator, our shared humanity, might not lead listeners to identify unjust structures, institutions, or policies that might produce these experiences. As we will return to in Chapters three and four, by stressing our similarities to the storyteller, these architectures might underestimate how we might not simply share their problems, but be part of them.

Berlant, in conversation with Jay Prosser in a recent issue of *Biography*, has talked about the way intimate publics might depoliticise. She commented:

> Intimate publics usually flourish to one side of politics, referring to historical subordinations without mobilising a fundamental activism with respect to them (think of illness publics, for example, which tend to spend most of their time moving between sharing expertise and survival stories, and less time mobilising against structural discrimination).
>
> (Berlant & Prosser, 2011, p. 184)

While the observation about illness narratives may well be true of the many "misery memoirs" that Couser (2012) observes emerging in the domain of literary non-fiction in recent years, we are not convinced that this is a fair assessment of the way that patient stories are used in professional education or service improvement contexts, as we will go on to discuss in more detail in Chapters three and four.

In contrast to Berlant's assertion here, many of the people we have spoken to in the course of researching this book emphatically stress the importance of framing and contextualising digital narratives. In particular, as we'll discuss in more detail in Chapters three and four, many of the people we've spoken to as we researched this book vehemently stress that digital stories don't speak for themselves. Amy Hill of Silence Speaks, for example, describing the workshops run by the organisation in conjunction with the Asian and Pacific Islander Wellness Center in the US, comments, "Frankly I don't think just showing them some touching stories is really going to do anything unless you show them, 'This is the issue, this is the data and this is what needs to be done about it'" (personal communication). However, outside the kinds of face-to-face encounters Hill is describing here, in online listening spaces, there are challenges in framing personal storytelling in this way, as we will show in the following case study.

Social media listening environments

The surge in enthusiasm in various forms of autobiographical digital storytelling – notably the digital storytelling movement – emerges at a period when the political focus on voice and new, cheaper computer and video technologies made multimedia participatory media possible and affordable (see for example, Dovey, 2000; Matthews, 2007). However, the appearance of multimedia participatory media platforms on the Web – Web 2.0 as it was once familiarly called – has outpaced formal digital storytelling projects. Perhaps unsurprisingly in the context of the boom in life narrative more generally (Couser, 2012), multimedia forms that draw from conventions of autobiographical storytelling – including vlogging – have come to be a key genre within online user-generated content, as a number of studies have suggested (i.e. Burgess & Green, 2009; Simonsen, 2011).

The emergence of social media hosts like Facebook and its competitors has made curating mediatised lives an everyday practice for many. The ease with which images and videos can now be collected, shared, and curated on these commercial social media sites means that even institutional sponsors of formal digital storytelling projects now frequently use host sites like YouTube or Vimeo to distribute or publicise their digital storytelling project. *Queensland Stories*, for instance, a collection of digital and video stories collected by the Queensland Library, has its own Vimeo channel, while Trusts within the Welsh NHS regularly use Twitter and YouTube to distribute and comment upon new stories.

While institutions involved in collecting digital stories have often wanted to maintain a certain amount of control over the platform they use and the data that might be generated from it, and have hence primarily used bespoke platforms, there has increasingly been a blurring of such listening infrastructures and pre-existing social media spaces. One of Valtysson's respondents, talking about a large-scale heritage digitisation project, commented:

> Facebook, Twitter, and Google are generally accepted platforms, and we need to make people aware of us, and it's through these commercial social media that we can reach out to users in easy and accessible ways. It's not like the portal would vanish if we put a link out on Facebook, and Facebook would close down. It's basically just similar to putting an advertisement in the paper.
>
> (Valtysson, 2015, p. 13)

This use of social media as a way of promoting an essentially separate space and the materials and objects hosted there could be seen as a rather conservative way of circulating multimodal digital stories. As Couldry and colleagues in their recent work on the extension of the digital story circle have suggested, digital storytelling and its publics have been expanded through platforms intended for sharing like Twitter, Facebook, Instagram, and Flickr (Clark, Couldry, & Stephansen, 2015). These forms open out notions of autobiographical narrative, challenging the notion of discrete and distinguishable stories.

Case study: Hypermodal and evolving digital stories

Photographer Angelo Merendino's cross-platform collection of stories of his wife's battle with breast cancer provides an excellent example of what we have previously referred to as a "reflective multimodal narrative" process (see Sunderland et al., 2015). Reflective multimodal narrative processes trace and adapt to the natural flows, diverse presentations, and evolution of personal stories over time. At the time of writing this book Merendino's publicly available story elements include a blog, art gallery exhibition of photographs,

Twitter account, the black and white photo documentary collection *The Battle We Didn't Choose – My Wife's Fight With Breast Cancer* (see http://m ywifesfightwithbreastcancer.com/photographs/), two TEDx talks *Photo Greater Than 1000* (https://www.youtube.com/watch?v=KeT221skphw) and *Community on Social Networks Sharing Experiences and Healing* (https://youtu.be/ GVH72spRYyM), and a Facebook site. Most elements of Merendino's story are available online for unlimited, un-negotiated, and untraceable sharing, recontextualisation, and remediation.

In his 2013 TEDx talk, Merendino (2013) explains that "words stopped working" as he and Jennifer tried to communicate to friends and family what daily life was like for them during Jennifer's cancer treatment and palliative care. Communication from family and friends had started to "drop off" as Jennifer's treatment and condition became more serious. Merendino said that he and Jennifer decided to move to his preferred "other" form of communication – photography – to try to communicate with friends and family what was happening and what the realities of cancer were. Merendino shared his photographs via a blog site which was intended originally for family and friends. The blog and associated story elements such as Merendino's photo documentary then went viral as listeners began to "tune in" from around the world. Merendino's listeners have included other women experiencing breast cancer and their families in particular. One woman contacted the couple through Angelo Merendino's blog and said that "because of Jen she faced her fears and scheduled a mammogram" (Merendino, 2013). In his TEDx talk of 2013 Merendino reflects "that's when we knew our story could help others" (Merendino, 2013).

In Merendino's case, a self-curated collection of story elements which arose from an intensely powerful and personal human experience have led to international recognition which culminated in the invitation to deliver two TEDx talks about his experiences of digital storytelling and cancer and being part of a networked community of healing through online storytelling. Merendino's two TEDx talks are delivered in personal narrative form and are now part of the broader meta-digital story he has co-created with Jennifer and their listeners. Merendino is storytelling about storytelling and it is available in digital multimodal form via YouTube (!). The blog site appears to be the central navigation point or perhaps "spine" of the meta-digital story with links and commentary about all other elements. The blog contains photo and text entries from before and after Jennifer Merendino's death from breast cancer (see http://mywifesfightwithbreastcancer.com/). For those new to Merendino's work, the TEDx talk delivered in the USA in 2013 offers an "up to that point" narrative of his and his wife's journey of storytelling through multimedia and multiple platforms for listening. Merendino's Facebook page documents the work he is now doing as a photo documentarist for other families facing terminal cancer diagnoses (see https://www.facebook.com/ Mywifesfightwithbreastcancer/). Merendino has also continued to make story "updates" to the Facebook page where he, for example, introduces his new girlfriend Jodi four years after the death of his wife Jennifer from breast cancer.

Other families and organisations have contacted Merendino over the time since his wife's death to invite him to join new photo documentary projects about breast cancer. These audience responses have become part of Merendino's ongoing story and storytelling. One of Merendino's latest projects, over four years since his own wife's death, has included photo documenting Holley and her family as Holley experiences breast cancer treatment. This is part of a broader initiative called *Story Half Told* which is an online community sponsored by pharmaceutical company Pfizer.

Theorising listening: the networked, hypermodal, evolving, and untethered story

A networked meta-digital story is one that emerges from the process of reflective multimodal narrative to include diverse but interrelated story elements across different listening infrastructures and environments. The networked meta-digital story both traces and documents the evolution of a person's

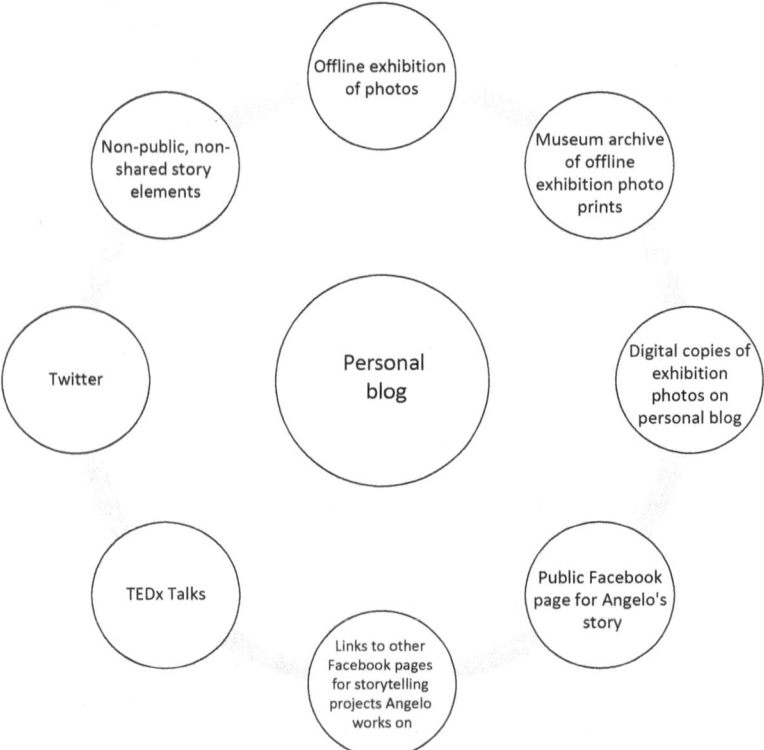

Figure 2.1 Angelo Merendino: example of a dynamic meta-digital story genre chain

narrative over time and space and allows for the inclusion of multiple media types in its formation. The potential audiences for stories are also multiplied through this type of cross-platform, multimodal, and cross-environment storytelling. In this way listeners can "stay with" and "follow" the storytellers as they grow, change, and experience. This is substantially different to a static presentation of a single digital story element where the storyteller's presentation of self is unable to naturally evolve over time as the "real" person evolves.

The ethical dimensions of this case study are edgy. They made themselves known to us in an embodied and sometimes uncomfortable "gut feeling" kind of way, flagging up the complexities of releasing personal story content into unfettered sharing and listening environments online. In this case study (see Figure 2.1) Angelo was simultaneously a co-storyteller, curator, host, witness, and caretaker of his and Jennifer's stories of breast cancer. It is not actually that easy to hear Jennifer's own "voice" in the resulting stories which raises ethical quandaries around vulnerability, consent, choice, and representation, among other things. No one could have ever predicted the way that this couple's initial representation of their own private experiences through a series of black and white photographs and blog posts then mutated and moved out into the world. No one could have predicted the recontextualisation and remediation of those stories as each new opportunity emerged both before and after Jennifer's death. Few would have predicted that this couple's story would be "taken up" within a broader and longer-term meta-narrative around metastatic breast cancer through the *Story Half Told* project or that pharmaceutical company Pfizer might become an institutional meta-orator for any of these women's and families' stories. When Jennifer gave her consent to be photographed in those stunning, powerful, and artistic ways could she have ever imagined that they would be discussed in this book after her death?

Take-aways for practitioners

- Consider the disadvantages as well as the advantages of "tethering" a story to its storyteller. Is the storyteller willing to have their story circulate into a range of listening environments if it is a way of meeting their aims in telling their story?
- Make sure you think about all of the possible uses that a story might finally have, and build all those uses into the consent form – especially if you don't have a multistage consent process.
- Caretakers for the stories may be as important as facilitators. Think about who will act as caretakers for funded projects after the project is finished.
- The full range of audiences for stories may not be anticipated at the beginning of the project. Think about how seeking consent for unanticipated uses of stories might be managed.
- Institutional memories about the story-making process can be short. How will the history of the story-making process and the people involved be preserved and made public?

- Is it possible to get "buy in" from PR and marketing staff within orga-nisations involved as commissioners or partners to ethical protocols around ways of using stories?
- Brokers may play an important role in the wider circulation of stories. Consider which institutions or individuals might play these roles?
- There are political implications to the ways you tag and categorise stories. Are the ways that readers navigate the site likely to subject them to the focusing illusion? Are there gains as well as losses in drawing out themes across stories rather than centring on case studies?
- Having a bespoke website for a collection of stories does not necessarily constrain the way those stories will circulate. Think about the ways that listeners and viewers might carry with them expectations from commercial media hosts.

Conclusion

There is no "correct" way to host or curate story collections. Decisions that are made about who can listen to stories, how they are organised, categorised, tagged, and searched, what platforms they are hosted on – the meta-oratory of these stories – all have implications for their meaning. The nature of listening environments, in particular, and the way they might frame individuals is easy to forget and has rarely been written about. The political as well as practical importance of the meta-oratory roles of listening curators, brokers, hosts, and caretakers shouldn't be underestimated, even in the case of online archives which might seem to "look after themselves". If increasingly listeners, viewers, and listening practices move across platforms, and there are doubts about the control that bespoke platforms seem to offer over the movement of stories, it is perhaps worth doing a careful assessment of the advantages and disadvantages of each type of platform, rather than assuming a bespoke platform will offer a more controlled or containable listening environment.

References

Alexandra, D. (2015). Are we listening yet? Participatory knowledge production through media practice: Encounters of political listening. In A. Gubrium, K. Harper, & M. Otanez (Eds.), *Participatory Visual and Digital Research in Action* (pp. 41–56). Abingdon: Left Coast Press.

Amundson, R. (2010). Quality of life, disability and hedonic psychology. *Journal for the Theory of Social Behaviour*, *40*(4), 374–392.

Berlant, L., & Prosser, J. (2011). Life writing and intimate publics: A conversation with Lauren Berlant. *Biography*, *34*(1), 180–187.

Bryson, K. (2012). The literacy myth in the Digital Archive of Literacy Narratives. *Computers and Composition*, *29*(3), 254–268.

Burgess, J. E. (2006). Hearing ordinary voices: Cultural studies, vernacular creativity and digital storytelling. *Continuum: Journal of Media and Cultural Studies*, *20*(2), 201–214. doi:10.1080/10304310600641737

Burgess, J., & Green, J. (2009). *YouTube: Online Video and Participatory Culture.* Cambridge: Polity Books.

Clark, W., Couldry, N., & Stephansen, H. (2015). Digital platforms and narrative exchange: Hidden constraints, emerging agency recognition. *New Media & Society, 17*(6), 919–938.

Clarke, M. (2014). Patient Voices: In celebration. In P. Hardy & T. Sumner (Eds.), *Cultivating Compassion: How Digital Storytelling is Transforming Healthcare* (pp. ix–xii). Chichester: Kingsham Press.

Collin, P. (2008). The internet, youth participation policies, and the development of young people's political identities in Australia. *Journal of Youth Studies, 11*(5), 527–542.

Comer, K., & Harker, M. (2015). The pedagogy of the Digital Archive of Literacy Narratives: A survey. *Computers and Composition, 35*, 65–85.

Copeland, S., & Miskelly, C. (2010). Making time for storytelling: The challenges of community building and activism in a rural locale. *Seminar.net – International Journal of Media, Technology and Lifelong Learning, 6*(2), 192–207.

Couldry, N. (2012). *Media, Society, World: Social Theory and Digital Media.* Cambridge: Polity Press.

Couser, G. T. (1997). *Recovering Bodies: Illness, Disability and Life Writing.* Madison: University of Wisconsin Press.

Couser, G. T. (2004). *Vulnerable Subjects: Ethics and Life Writing.* Ithaca, NY: Cornell University Press.

Couser, G. T. (2012). *Memoir: An Introduction.* London: Oxford University Press.

Couser, G. T. (2014, March). Narrating disability inside and outside the clinic: Or, beyond empathy. Seminar conducted at Liverpool Hope University College, Centre for Culture and Disability Studies, Liverpool.

Deschamp, P. (2009). *Wild Animals in Skips.* Retrieved from http://1000voices.edu.au/wild-animals-skips

Dovey, J. (2000). *Freakshow: First Person Media and Factual Television.* London: Pluto Press.

Dreher, T. (2012). A partial promise of voice: Digital storytelling and the limit of listening. *Media International Australia Incorporating Culture and Policy: Quarterly Journal of Media Research and Resources, 142*, 157–166.

Dush, L. (2013). The ethical complexities of sponsored digital storytelling. *International Journal of Cultural Studies, 16*(6), 627–640.

Fuchs, C. (2014). *Social Media: A Critical Introduction.* London: Sage.

Gubrium, A., Hill, A., & Flicker, S. (2014). A situated practice of ethics for participatory visual and digital methods in public health practice: A focus on digital storytelling. *American Journal of Public Health, 104*(9), e1–e9. doi: 10.2105/AJPH.2013.301310

Hardy, P., & Sumner, T. (Eds.) (2014). *Cultivating Compassion: How Digital Storytelling is Transforming Healthcare.* Chichester: Kingsham Press.

Harrison, S., & Mort, M. (1998). Which champions? Which people? Public and user involvement in health care as a technology of legitimation. *Social Policy and Administration, 32*(1), 60–70.

Hartley, J. (2007, May). The problems of expertise and scalability in self-made media: Lessons from digital storytelling in Australia. 57th Annual International Communication Association (ICA) Conference, San Francisco, CA.

Hessler, B., & Lambert, J. (2017, forthcoming). Threshold concepts of digital storytelling: Naming what we know about storywork. In Y. Nordkvelle, G. Jamissen,

P. Hardy, & H. Pleasants (Eds.), *Digital Storytelling in Higher Education: International Perspectives*. Melbourne: Palgrave Macmillan.

Juliano, L., & Srinivasan, R. (2012). Tagging it: Considering how ontologies limit the reading of identity. *International Journal of Cultural Studies, 15*(5), 615–627.

Lambert, J. (2009). Where it all started: The Centre for Digital Storytelling in California. In J. Hartley & K. McWilliam (Eds.), *Story Circle: Digital Storytelling around the World* (pp. 79–90). Chichester, UK: Wiley.

Lemke, J. L. (2002). Travels in hypermodality. *Visual Communication, 1*(3), 299–325.

Lessig, L. (1999). *Code and Other Laws of Cyberspace*. New York: Basic Books.

Lewis, K. & Matthews, N. (2017, forthcoming). The afterlife of *Capture Wales*: Digital stories and their listening publics. In T. Jenkins & M. Dunham (Eds.), *Digital Storytelling: Form and Content*. London: Palgrave.

Locock, L., Robert, G., Boaz, A., Vougioukalou, S., Shuldham, C., Fielden, J., Ziebland, S., Gager, M., Tollyfield, R., & Pearcey, J. (2014). Using a national archive of patient experience narratives to promote local patient-centered quality improvement: An ethnographic process evaluation of 'accelerated' experience-based co-design. *Journal of Health Services Research & Policy, 19*(4), 200–207.

McKee, A. (2011). YouTube versus the National Film and Sound Archive: Which is the more useful resource for historians of Australian television? *Television and New Media, 12*(2), 154–173.

Matthews, N. (2007). Confessions to a new public: Video Nation shorts. *Media, Culture and Society, 29*(3), 435–448. doi: 10.1177/0163443707076184

Matthews, N., & Sunderland, N. (2013). Digital life-story narratives as data for policy makers and practitioners: Thinking through methodologies for large-scale multimedia qualitative datasets. *Journal of Broadcasting & Electronic Media, 57*(1), 97–114.

Merendino, A. (2013). *Photo Greater than 1000: Angelo Merendino at TEDxUSU* [YouTube]. Retrieved from https://www.youtube.com/watch?v=KeT221skphw

Mitchell, D. (2015). *The Biopolitics of Disability: Neoliberalism, Ablenationalism, and Peripheral Embodiment*. Ann Arbor: University of Michigan Press.

Poletti, A. (2011). Coaxing an intimate public: Life narrative in digital storytelling. *Continuum: Journal of Media & Cultural Studies, 25*(1), 73–83.

Polk, E. (2010). Folk media meets digital technology for sustainable social change: A case study of the Center for Digital Storytelling. *Global Media Journal, 10*(17), n.p.

Shilton, K. (2015). Anticipatory ethics for a future Internet: Analyzing values during the design of an internet infrastructure. *Science and Engineering Ethics, 21*(1), 1–18.

Simonsen, T. M. (2011). Categorising YouTube. *MedieKultur, 27*(51), 72–93.

Sonke Gender Justice (n.d.). *Digital Storytelling Project: Using Narrative and Participatory Media to Explore the Links between Gender, Violence, and HIV and AIDS in South Africa. A Case Study*. Retrieved from http://www.genderjustice.org.za/publication/silence-speaks/

Sunderland, N., Bristed, H., Gudes, O., Boddy, J., & Da Silva, M. (2012). What does it feel like to live here? Exploring sensory ethnography as a collaborative methodology for investigating social determinants of health in place. *Health and Place, 18*(5), 1056–1067.

Sunderland, N., Chenoweth, L., Matthews, N., & Ellem, K. (2015). 1000 Voices: Reflective online multimodal narrative inquiry as a research methodology for disability research. *Qualitative Social Work, 14*(1), 48–64. doi: 10.1177/1473325014523818

Sunderland, N., Kendall, E., & Catalano, T. (2009). Missing discourses: Concepts of joy and happiness in disability. *Disability and Society, 24*(6), 703–714. doi: 10.1080/09687590903160175

Tacchi, J., & Grubb, B. (2007). The case of the e-tuktuk. *Media International Australia incorporating Culture and Policy, 125*, 71–82.

Tacchi, J., Watkins, J., & Keerthirathne, K. (2009). Participatory content creation: Voice, communication and development. *Development in Practice, 19*(4), 573–584.

Thumim, N. (2007). *Mediating Self-Representations: Tensions Surrounding Ordinary People's Participation in Public Sector Projects.* London: School of Economics and Political Science.

Thumim, N. (2009). Everyone has a story to tell: Mediation and self-representation in two UK institutions. *International Journal of Cultural Studies, 12*(6), 617–638. doi: 10.1177/1367877909342494

Valtysson, B. (2015). From policy to platform: The digitization of Danish cultural heritage. *International Journal of Cultural Policy.* doi: 10.1080/10286632.2015.1084300

Van Dijck, J. (2013). *The Culture of Connectivity: A Critical History of Social Media.* Oxford: Oxford University Press.

Vivienne, S., & Burgess, J. (2012). The digital storyteller's stage: Queer everyday activists negotiating privacy and publicness. *Journal of Broadcast and Electronic Media, 56*(3), 362–377.

Wang, X. (2013). *A genre theory perspective on digital storytelling* (Doctoral dissertation). Nashville, TN: Vanderbilt University.

Wilson, D. K., Hutson, S. P., & Wyatt, T. H. (2015). Exploring the role of digital storytelling in pediatric oncology patients' perspectives regarding diagnosis. *SAGE Open, 5*(1). doi: 10.1177/2158244015572099.

Yea, S. (2015). Girls on film: Affective politics and the creation of an intimate anti-trafficking public in Singapore through film screenings. *Political Geography, 45*, 45–54.

3   Listening in professional education

In this chapter we visit our first specific context for listening to digital stories: professional health education. Many of us who are excited by digital storytelling as an educational strategy have encouraged our students to make their own stories and use them as a basis for reflection and metacognition – thinking about thinking and critically reflecting on professional roles and behaviours. In the first part of the chapter, we briefly examine why student-generated digital stories are a popular use of digital storytelling in higher education and the ideas that underpin this approach. In the second part of the chapter we turn our focus to a perhaps less commonly considered use of digital storytelling: that is, getting students and professionals to listen to health service users' stories. The case study material for this chapter focuses on dementia care education. We outline the ways that "classic" digital storytelling has been used for dementia care education in two projects: Rosie Stenhouse and Patient Voices' *Dangling Conversations* project at the University of Abertay in Scotland and the South Australia and Northern Territory's Dementia Training Study Centre's *Visual Stories* collection. Our primary aim here is to unpack and theorise some of the strategies that trainers and teachers have used to get learners to listen to others' stories, and to reflect on some of the practical and ethical challenges of using these materials as teaching tools.

Digital storytelling in professional education settings

Digital storytelling has been widely discussed in the literature on education (McWilliam, 2008). Community arts and community education was the birthplace of digital storytelling, but mediated storytelling has also been adapted in formal education from primary school through to adult and professional education (Lambert, 2009; McWilliam, 2008). Teachers report that digital storytelling can serve a number of important functions in the classroom. Reflecting and talking about your own experiences can enhance literacy (Kajder, 2004) and digital literacies in particular; engage and motivate learners (Sadik, 2008; Smeda, Dakich, & Sharda, 2014); and help develop research skills (Robin, 2006). While some, particularly those working in the field of medical education, note the instructional possibilities of teacher-authored case studies or teaching materials (D'Alessandro, Lewis, & D'Alessandro, 2004; Pullman, Bethune, & Duke, 2005; Robin, 2006), most research on the use of digital storytelling in higher education emphasises the value of learners telling stories about their own experiences (Brushwood Rose & Low, 2014; Kearney, 2011; Kocaman-Karoglu, 2016; Lowenthal, 2009; Sadik, 2008; Thompson-Long & Hall, 2017).

Rina Benmayor (2008) describes digital storytelling as a "signature pedagogy" in the humanities because it prompts:

> active learning process that engages the cultural assets, experiences and funds of knowledge that students bring to the classroom. It is also a self-reflexive and recursive process that helps students to make important intellectual (theorizing) and personally transformative moves.
>
> (p. 189)

In education contexts, the critique of educational authority emerging from progressive education theory in the 1960s and 1970s has led – at least in the longer term – to an increasing focus on active, student-centred learning. Critical pedagogy approaches, drawing on the work of Paulo Freire, for instance, stress the value of the existing knowledge of students and the problems of a hierarchical relationship between teacher and student. Freirian approaches to learning query "banking" approaches to teaching that view teachers as authoritative knowers and learners as empty vessels, passively absorbing "deposits" of information.

This approach to learning has been influential in the way digital storytelling has been conceptualised as an educational tool. Amy Hill, co-founder of Silence Speaks, explains how Freire's perspectives on learning have shaped the organisation's approach. Silence Speaks shares Freire's concern with "the development of critical consciousness, a precursor to action for social change" (Hill, 2008, p. 50). Such processes, she suggests, "must begin with close examination of one's own experience in an unjust social and political context" (Hill, 2008; see also Hessler & Lambert, 2017). Reflection on your own individual socially and politically shaped experiences is key to political change in this account.

The enthusiasm with which digital storytelling has been taken up in informal and community education reflects the link between the "movement" and the idea of progressive social change. Daniel Meadows (2003) has argued that digital storytelling should be seen fundamentally as a community media practice, with connections to folk traditions and oral history (see also McWilliam, 2008; Polk, 2010). In community settings storytelling has been valued for encouraging marginalised groups to articulate and reflect on their own experience in ways that build diverse literacies, confidence, and a sense of community (Hull & Katz, 2006, p. 6). Digital storytelling seems, on the one hand, like a natural approach to take when working with marginalised young people who may already have a familiarity with but perhaps limited access to digital tools (Burgess, 2006; Podkalicka, 2009; Wexler, Eglinton, & Gubrium, 2014). On the other, it has also been reached for as a key strategy for closing the "digital divide" and supporting learning for people who may not be familiar with digital technologies, or not have ready access to them, such as older or homeless people (Brushwood Rose & Low, 2014). While such programs have often been framed as learning opportunities, such informal learning has been seen in part as building social capacity and generating a sense of community. Often, learning, then, has been seen as just one, and often not the most important, purpose of telling personal multimedia stories.

Despite the unambiguous origins of digital storytelling in emancipatory political frameworks, the ways in which such progressive educational approaches have played out in further and higher education settings are complex and politically multivalent. As Kevin Robins and Frank Webster note in their book, *The Times of the Technoculture* (Robins & Webster, 1999), in the UK, aspirations for student-centred and active learning only gained purchase in further and higher education in the early 1980s. Ideas about student-centred learning found a warm reception in the UK; at the time a Conservative British government was encouraging the uptake of market logics in public services of all kinds. The notion of the active, autonomous, and self-managing learner, emerging from progressive critiques of conservative, hierarchical conceptions of learning, converged with a view of education as offering a service to choosy consumers. Traditional teacher-centred pedagogies in this moment were seen by both neoliberal conservatives and educational progressives as examples of vested interests protecting unjust hierarchies of power. The figure of the autonomous learner, bringing their own history and choices to education, fits well with digital storytelling as a pedagogic strategy for allowing students to record and reflect on their own unique experiences. Equally, the stress in many digital storytelling projects on the digital literacy skills that learners will develop through telling their stories fits, perhaps a little more uneasily, with the emphasis on skills in this new paradigm of education, with its stress on the importance of retooling university education to better prepare graduates for the employment market.

While we have found a few examples of teachers using digital storytelling as an opportunity to get students to listen to the narratives of others, particularly in nursing education (see for instance, Christiansen, 2011; Gidman, 2012; Davis, 2011), this is very much a minority practice. Overwhelmingly, digital storytelling is used in classrooms and in professional training contexts as an opportunity for learners to tell their own stories and learn by reflecting on them (Anderson, 2017; Hardy, 2017; Thompson-Long & Hall, 2017). This is equally true in the field of health, as Carol Haigh and Pip Hardy note in their review of storytelling in health education (Haigh & Hardy, 2011). Listening, where it appears, happens primarily as students in the same group listen to each other in preparing stories, or towards the end of the project when completed stories are shared.

Why, then, have teachers using storytelling as an approach tended to focus on telling rather than listening? We will suggest that the powerful hold of reflection in contemporary thinking about education, and particularly the notion of reflective practice, have played a role. In order to use digital story-telling in alternative ways in higher education, we'll suggest we might need to broaden the ways we understand reflexivity, and think more closely about the role of listening within reflection. Rather than relying on the inherent power of the activity of making a digital story to prompt reflection, we will be looking to the ways teachers and trainers have tried to scaffold and frame listening in order to try to prompt reflection.

Student-generated digital storytelling and the reflective practitioner

The effectiveness of both autobiographical storytelling and more specifically digital storytelling has been described in terms of its power to prompt reflection (Benmayor, 2008; Conle, 2000; Hardy, 2017; Jenkins & Lonsdale, 2007; Pfahl & Wiessner, 2007, Rossiter & Garcia, 2010; Thompson-Long & Hall, 2017). The ideal of reflection has become an unquestioned aim of many education programs. The key research question in these traditions is not whether reflection should be the aim, but how the curriculum can be shaped to make sure learners become reflective practitioners (Barrett, 2006; Jenkins & Lonsdale, 2007; Sandars & Murray, 2009). Indeed, Melaine Coward (2011) has described nursing students in particular as suffering from "reflection fatigue" given the number of assessments they are required to undertake that push them towards such activities.

Our aim here is not to critique this approach. We agree that metacognitive skills – thinking about thinking – are critical tools for learning, and particularly for making sense of, and trying to intervene in, unjust social relationships. However, we are interested in extending and enriching this emphasis on reflection by exploring ways in which listening to *others'* stories might be used as a route towards learning.

As Janice McDrury and Maxine Alterio note in their work on storytelling as a tool in higher education (McDrury & Alterio, 2002), there's much debate over the exact definition of reflection, but one common feature of a range of definitions is their focus on the self and one's own experiences (p. 21). A well-known formulation of reflection is that of David Boud, Rosemary Keogh, and David Walker: "reflection in the context of learning is a generic term for those intellectual and affective abilities in which individuals engage to explore their experiences in order to lead to new understandings and appreciations" (Boud, Keogh, & Walker, 1985, p. 19). We would argue that the great value placed on learning through reflection on one's own experiences makes the idea of using others' autobiographical stories as a source of information and possible transformation seem a less than obvious pedagogical tool. Yet many writers on reflection as a tool for learning suggest that at its deepest and most critical levels, reflection involves questioning your own assumptions and perspectives and seeing events in a range of different ways (Coulson & Harvey, 2012; Mann, Gordon, & MacLeod, 2009; McDrury & Alterio, 2002). While the sharing of stories within the classroom may be very valuable, medical students listening to other medical students' stories, for example, are likely to hear something very different from medical students required to listen to stories from their patients (see for instance, Christiansen, 2011; Gidman, 2012).

Our conversations with facilitators and teachers using digital storytelling to prompt learning from others suggest that reflection is indeed an important part of this process. However, to share methods for making such stories intelligible and "listenable" we need to move on from a pedagogy and practice that focuses on reflection on one's own life narrative, towards one that considers reflection on your own life as part of the process of listening to others' stories. What we aim to do in this chapter is explore the ways in which this might be done. We want to move beyond the assumption that, because digital stories emerge from storytellers' deep processes of reflection, they necessarily prompt reflection in their audiences (Haigh & Hardy, 2011). Rather we want to consider what strategies might work to prompt learners to critically reflect in the light of listening to other people's stories, and what challenges are posed in trying to make other people's autobiographical stories "listenable".

Listening as passive? A counter-example: the Clinical Leadership program of the UK's Royal College of Nursing

We observed in Chapter one that listening as a process has been neglected in media and cultural theory over the past forty years in comparison to voice. In the context of the use of digital storytelling as a pedagogy, this elision of listening may be connected to the association of listening with more conventional learning strategies. As we have argued, digital storytelling has often been seen as a progressive strategy to encourage active, student-centred, experiential learning in stark contrast to the perceived passivity associated with more conventional modes of teaching, such as the lecture, with listening seen as a part of that tradition. This equation of listening with passivity and speaking with activity, it has been recently argued, reflects deep-seated assumptions within Western political traditions around democracy and choice. Speaking up in public spaces has been associated with the workings of democracy since at least John Stuart Mill, while, at least until recently, listening has rarely been discussed as a key component of democracy (Mondal, 2016).

One influential exception has been the UK Royal College of Nursing's Clinical Leadership program. A key element of this training and accreditation program has incorporated collection and analysis of patient stories. This is a key instance of the use of storytelling associated with professional education in health in the UK and underpins the use of stories in other contexts, notably, the use of storytelling, including the use of digital storytelling for service improvement in the NHS Wales 1000 Lives project, as discussed in Chapter four.

In 2001 the UK's Royal College of Nursing and the National Health System Leadership centre introduced a third phase of a clinical leadership program which had been running since 1995, which aimed to produce "self-aware leaders, motivated to produce real improvements in clinical practice and to establish direction and purpose, to inspire and motivate their teams" (Large, Macleod, Kitson, & Cunningham, 2005, p. 8). A key element of this third phase was the collection of a number of patient stories by nurses undertaking the program. Collection of patient stories is framed in the program as a patient-focused intervention, alongside the observation of care. The aim of collecting these stories, which are recorded as spoken oral narratives, is to document experiences of care with a view to service improvement.

Participants in the program were paired up in such a way that stories were not collected by staff in their own area of work. Each pair collected six patient stories and analysed them for themes of valued and less valued experiences of care, which were then visually mapped. Elements of narrative were sometimes incorporated into this mapping – for instance, the onset of illness or injury, the arrival of the patient in hospital, their experience there, and their discharge from hospital (Green & Davies, 2009). Themes and issues were discussed first with another clinical leader and then with a multidisciplinary team. In theory, if not always in practice (Large et al., 2005, p. 32), an action plan was made by that team to identify changes in practice in that clinical area. The Royal College of Nursing (2004) toolkit for patient-centred interventions stresses the importance of ensuring the patients telling their stories feel they are listened to. For instance, it suggests that, if a patient mentions being cold at night, or being bothered by a noisy door, or the need to contact social services, these matters should be followed up immediately (Large et al., 2005, p. 45).

While this example of listening to patient stories did not take the form of multimedia digital storytelling, it offers an unusual instance of the use of story collection and listening to stories as a key part of professional education. The 2005 evaluation of the clinical leadership program emphasised the different experience of listening to such stories, by comparison to the taking of a clinical history. The toolkit for facilitators of the clinical leadership program emphasises the fact that "the content of each interview is led by the individual patient/client" (Royal College of Nursing, 2004, p. 7.24). This focus on a patient-centred approach is shared with Storycenter's approach to digital storytelling discussed in Chapter one.

In some respects, the activities required by the Royal College of Nursing sidestep the contradiction between the conventional assumption of listening as passive and student-initiated storytelling as active. Requiring nurses in positions of clinical leadership to collect and transcribe patient stories as a precursor and component of listening to the stories, reflecting and discussing them, and making changes to practice in conjunction with work colleagues reframes listening as both active and reflective.

This long-standing training scheme has shaped the ways in which stories have been collected and listened to in the British NHS. The idea that nurses are the natural collectors of stories has almost become a commonplace in health care settings in the UK. In fact, the idea that it is nurses who are most likely to collect stories has become so taken-for-granted in the British health care system that listening brokers like patient experience managers in the NHS arguing for the importance of patient stories have had to emphasise that it is possible for others to take on this role (personal communication, patient experience managers, Wales). This exemplar of listening to patient stories also shaped the systematic approaches to collecting and using digital stories as part of service improvement in the Welsh NHS, as we will discuss in detail in Chapter four.

Case study: Listening to digital stories in dementia education

We want to step away now from the assumption that listening is a passive process, aligned with conservative pedagogies. To help us think through ways of using autobiographical narratives in professional education, we want to outline the way digital life stories have been used in two very different contexts to enhance dementia care. In Scotland, the Patient Voices project team (see Pilgrim Projects, 2016) worked with Rosie Stenhouse, then at the University of Abertay, to develop a suite of "classic" digital stories by people with dementia that could be used in undergraduate nursing education. The stories were made available initially on the university website along with teaching and learning materials, and continue to be available on the *Patient Voices* site. Rosie Stenhouse and Jo Tait from Patient Voices have written about their experiences of developing and using the stories, and we have drawn on their accounts here. In a very different project, in Australia, as part of a government-funded network of training centres, the South Australian and Northern Territory Dementia Training Centre, run by the Alzheimer's Association, developed a collection of digital stories – *Visual Stories* – some made by people with dementia and some by carers or family members. These stories were used in a range of training contexts, from short half-day training sessions with under-graduate medical and allied health students, to fee-for-service training for aged care workers in their place of work, to initial training for long-term unem-ployed people seeking to work in aged care. The DVD of the stories was also distributed Australia-wide, with evidence from our survey of users suggesting many recipients used the collection to train staff in their own place of work.

The following case study was prepared using documentary and multimedia evidence available in the public sphere in addition to documents provided by the SA and NT Dementia Care Study Centre and the Dementia Centre at Stirling University. It was also supplemented by focus groups, an online survey, and in-depth interviews conducted between 2012 and 2016. Formal interviews were conducted under an approved ethics protocol via Macquarie University. Those we interviewed for this case study have only been identified based on their express request to be so.

The health educators we spoke to who had chosen to use digital life stories as a teaching tool acknowledged the value of the face-to-face encounters with patients that they might replace. One dementia educator we interviewed commented:

That's just invaluable having someone right there that you can touch, but the reality of that is getting that person. Again it's got to be the right person, right time. That's a hard gig ... there's not a lot of people that can do that consistently and they will wear out, as we all do.

(personal communication, dementia care trainer, Australia)

Trainers articulated concerns not just about the availability of self-advocates but expressed concern about the potential vulnerability of people, particularly those with progressive cognitive impairments, speaking to learners about their experience. One worry that trainers shared was that self-advocates might disclose information that they later regretted, for example.

Listening to digital stories by people with dementia or their families was seen as a potentially valuable tool for training staff for a range of different reasons. In particular it was seen as offering an opportunity to challenge preconceptions around the condition. As one trainer we spoke to commented, "they've already got the picture, it's an old decrepit person in a nursing home, that's who you're talking about" (personal communication, dementia care trainer, Australia). She went on to say, "you show them someone that's quite young and still talking very well ... you stop that and say to people what do you think? Quite often the first thing that people say is 'they're very young'. And it's like 'oh gosh, I'm that age'." Digital stories featuring people with younger-onset dementia were particularly memorable for the small number of people who responded to our online survey.

The rich, experiential, and visual information in digital stories was seen as particularly helpful in motivating learners, especially those who are in the process of retraining or have difficulty accessing written material in English. One trainer noted: "if somebody has had no experience in the area whatsoever, if I get up and talk too much about it I'm going to lose them and they're not going to follow what I'm saying, whereas if they can see it, it's a lot more helpful to them" (personal communication, dementia care trainer, Australia). The realism of digital stories was also flagged up as an advantage of these resources, an effect noted in the evaluation of the online resources of the *Telling Stories* website, hosted by the UK NHS's National Genetics and Genomics Education Centre, and discussed in Chapter two (Burke, 2008, p. 10). A Queensland-based trainer working in aged care who responded to our survey on digital stories commented along similar lines: "real stories have more of an impact than just those who talk statistics." In the same survey a clinical nurse consultant working in a hospital in South Australia suggested that digital stories were preferable to scenarios or fiction-based texts because of their realism, including their depiction of emotions (online survey).

Digital storytelling and person-centred care

A key advantage of digital storytelling in dementia-training sessions, according to trainers we spoke to, was its fit with a key, some might say "all-pervading", approach to dementia care education: person-centred care (Brooker, 2003, p. 215). Indeed, person-centred care has had an influence across health care contexts since the early 1990s (Jefferies & Horsfall, 2013; McKeown, Clarke, Ingleton, Ryan, & Repper, 2010; Nay, Bird, Edvardsson, Fleming, & Hill, 2009; Nolan, Davies, Brown, Keady, & Nolan, 2004; Schwind, Lindsay, Coffey, Morrison, & Mildon, 2014). There is a convergence between the philosophy of digital storytelling, with its emphasis on individual experience and the uniqueness of the individual voice, and underpinning values of person-centred care. Tom Kitwood's (1997) work expanding on this concept has been particularly influential in dementia education (O'Connor et al., 2007; Sheard, 2008; Walsh, 2006). Kitwood (1997) argues for a shift in dementia care, from a biomedical understanding of dementia and a focus on treating health problems, to a concern with the person with dementia. He emphasises that people with dementia must be "regarded as persons in the full sense ... recognized, welcomed, embraced and heard" (p. 133). He advocates for transformations in aged care institutions and changes in the way professional and family carers communicate with and consider people with dementia to enable a "new" culture of care to emerge (Kitwood, 1997, p. 143).

Kitwood stresses the importance of validation in dementia care. Validation, he suggests:

> is to make strong or robust; to validate the experience of another is to accept the reality and power of that experience, and hence its "subjective truth". The heart of the matter is acknowledging the reality of a person's emotions and feelings ... Validation involves a high degree of empathy, attempting to understand a person's entire frame of reference.
>
> (Kitwood, 1997, p. 91)

It's clear how this emphasis on the person with dementia's individual experience, and the need to cultivate empathy, fits well with the emphasis on individual voice and compassion in digital storytelling. Dawn Brooker (2003) defines person-centred care in dementia in terms of four elements – valuing the person with dementia, creating a positive social environment, "treating people as individuals", and "looking at the world from the perspective of the person with dementia" (p. 216). These last two features, in particular, fit very clearly with the philosophy of the digital storytelling movement.

Life story work in dementia care settings

The ethical and practical challenges of people with advanced dementia participating in digital storytelling workshops have meant that there have only been a few projects where "classic" digital stories have been collected (Stenhouse & Tait, 2014; Stenhouse, Tait, Hardy, & Sumner, 2013). However reminiscence therapies and life story work have become widely used in dementia care settings (Gridley et al., 2015; Gridley, 2016). Making life story books or recording reminiscences about the past can be a meaningful and enjoyable activity for people whose memory of recent events may not be as intact as their recall of the long-distant past. The books or recordings that come out of these activities are viewed as potentially useful information for professional caregivers, especially as the disease progresses and storytellers become less able to give an account of their own background, experiences, interests, and preferences. As one trainer remarked in conversation with us, "Learning about a person's past helps our understanding or interpretation of present behaviour" (personal communication, dementia care trainer, Scotland). Recent research has explored the practical value of life story narratives in the process of care transitions – from living at home to being looked after in a nursing home for instance (Gridley et al., 2015; Gridley, 2016)

Life story work is also an important educational strategy built into programs and learning materials to train people to work in dementia care. In looking through the kinds of textbooks and learning packages that have been developed to help people work in aged care settings, it is evident that the idea of reflecting on one's own life experiences as a route to understanding the experiences of others is a key teaching technique. The University of Stirling's *Best Practice in Dementia Care* training package for domiciliary staff includes a number of exercises involving writing short accounts of aspects of the learner's own life and reflecting on them. For instance, it asks learners to "Think about what makes you different from a close friend or colleague. Write down your responses below" (University of Stirling, 2012, p. 9). The shared experiences of workers and those they worked with are stressed in these texts – for instance, the shared experience of forgetfulness, or being unable to find the right words. A unique and individual life story is also emphasised as another shared ground. "People with dementia have a similar collection of life experiences to you and I. Seeing the individual and not the dementia means focusing on the characteristics that make each one of us unique and different" (University of Stirling, 2012, p. 9). Very similar exercises reflecting on what makes you an individual and comparing your individuality to your knowledge of the patients you work with are part of many teaching guides for people training staff to work with people with dementia (Mace, Coons, & Weaverdyck, 2005; Walsh, 2006).

The central themes of these training materials are the bedrock of shared human experiences, needs, and values, and the importance of stories of individual lives as ways into the shared experience of uniqueness. The similarities between those caring for people with dementia and those being cared for are often stressed in training sessions as well. One Scottish trainer, for instance, stressed her emphasis in training that "interpreting the person's behaviour successfully involves putting ourselves in their shoes and asking what they might be trying to communicate" (personal communication, dementia care trainer, Scotland). Feeling empathy with the person with dementia, according to many training texts, is seen as key for professional carers effectively to support them (Mace et al., 2005, p. 48:2).

Testimonial injustice

The philosopher Miranda Fricker uses two concepts that are helpful in making sense of how life story telling, including digital storytelling, has been used to shape listening in dementia care education: testimonial injustice and testimonial sensibilities. Havi Carel and Ian Kidd (2014) have shown how Fricker's ideas can be used to think through the relationship between professionals and patients in healthcare contexts. Fricker (2003) suggests that a fundamental form of social injustice is what she calls "testimonial injustice", that is, when the listener's prejudices make them disinclined to believe what a person has to say (p. 154). She discusses the way racism and sexism, for example, play a significant part in shaping which stories are viewed as plausible and which are viewed as suspect. She argues that to overcome such testimonial injustice, listeners need to develop new rules of thumb about the statements of particular types of speakers – what she calls "testimonial sensibilities". These "testimonial sensibilities" operate, she suggests, below the radar of conscious decision-making, serving more as a feeling or instinct for whether a person is believable.

We suggest here that life story has become so important in dementia care education because of the way it promises to help reshape the testimonial sensibilities of workers and carers. One of the key shifts in thinking that dementia educators who talked to us were keen to promote through their training was the way the behaviour of people with dementia was interpreted by their professional carers. "When you train, what they want more than anything from you as an educator, the biggest thing they want is, 'Tell me how to manage these behaviours, just tell me how to manage them'" – as one Australian dementia trainer told us (personal communication). But the emphasis in training was reinterpreting such "challenging" or difficult behaviours as forms of communication.

One dementia care trainer in Scotland explained why people come to training sessions:

> people would have registered interest because they have awful problems – what they call "managing behaviour". [We] try and change their sort of reference point and get them to think of ... challenging behaviours, aggressive behaviours as signs of distress and so we emphasise communication and trying to encourage people to understand what the person is trying to communicate, and then they can support them better once they understand that. And life stories, that's essential to that because it's about knowing the person.
>
> (personal communication)

The idea of "testimonial sensibility" is again helpful here. Carel and Kidd (2014) describe various forms of testimonial injustice – not being heard, not being acknowledged, or one's statements being heard and acknowledged but not acted upon (p. 532). But what the dementia trainers we spoke to were concerned about was an even more fundamental kind of testimonial injustice – when a person's attempt at communication may not be recognised as communication at all (Carel & Kidd, 2014, p. 532). While many people with dementia are powerful self-advocates, as the work on person-centred care for people with dementia points out, often "behaviours that challenge" should be read instead as responses to unmet needs or attempts to communicate those needs (Keady & Jones, 2010, p. 28).

Listening to digital stories, then, has been used as one strategy of dementia trainers in trying to encourage professional carers to see the person who may be trying to communicate, rather than a person exhibiting symptoms of a disease. These particular moments of listening are intended to help reshape the ways that staff might be oriented to listen in general.

Dangling conversations: online digital life stories in person-centred care

An important example of the use of digital storytelling in dementia care education to achieve this person-centred focus is the *Dangling Conversations* learning resource developed by Dr Rosie Stenhouse (n.d.), then based at Abertay University, in conjunction with Patient Voices. Patient Voices were commissioned to work with people with dementia to develop a series of classic digital stories for use as part of nurse education. The freely available "dementia learning package" describes its aim as to:

> engage the audience with the storyteller's experience. You are encouraged to watch each story and reflect on what the story makes you feel and think ... You should also think about how these reflections would influence how you work with people with dementia.
>
> (Stenhouse, n.d.)

While the package as a whole is framed by the diagnostic label of "dementia", the individual stories are labelled in a way that highlights the past and present skills, professions, and enthusiasms of the storyteller (Stenhouse, n.d.). The introduction to the package notes that, "The digital story making method let participants tell the story that they chose and did not demand that people talked directly about their experience of dementia." Stenhouse emphasises the focus of the stories on articulating voices of the people with dementia. She notes that she chose to commission Patient Voices because "the storytelling and story creation was patient controlled, fitting with my desire to open up spaces for the voices of the participants (rather than researchers) to be heard" (Stenhouse & Tait, 2014).

The fact that most of these stories don't explicitly or overtly thematise the experience of dementia at first troubled Stenhouse. Concerns about the "teachability" of the autobiographical narratives of people with dementia have been shared by others using these stories for training. However, she concludes, "I think they do the job because the audience hears the story knowing that the storyteller has dementia. That's what makes them powerful, because it is not the dementia that's presented, it's the person" (Stenhouse & Tait, 2014). Stenhouse and Tait (2014) suggest that these stories encourage students to engage emotionally as well as cognitively with the experiences of storytellers.

The learning resources around *Dangling Conversations* mirror this focus on reflection and personhood. The questions for reflection posed around the films include questions that prompt interrogation of students' preconceptions or expectations – for instance, "How did this picture of Aileen fit with your ideas about someone with dementia?" or "Does anything surprise you about Alec's story?" Students are encouraged to make notes under three headings after listening to each story: "What the story made me think. What the story made me feel. Ideas for how I can use this knowledge when working with people with dementia." The learning materials associated with the *Dangling Conversations* are open ended. Some of these prompt students to consider their professional practice and in particular to think through how their own practice might enhance the lives of people like the storytellers. For instance: "What kind of approach might help you engage with Alec if you were nursing him in a hospital setting?"

Stenhouse and her colleagues, in their evaluation of the *Dangling Conversations* collection of digital stories, found that these stories did indeed encourage their students to see "the person behind the illness" (Stenhouse & Tait, 2014). Feedback from students attending the Dementia Training Study Centre (DTSC) in Adelaide included similar comments about their training. A fifth-year medical student commented after his training, which included watching digital stories, that he learned that "patients are people with a history & something to lose, especially in dementia" (personal communication). A number of people working in aged care settings or hospitals in training roles who responded to our qualitative survey about "Visual Stories", the collection of digital stories used at the DTSC in Adelaide, described digital life stories as a valuable strategy for "holistic person centred care" (survey response, clinical practice consultant, South Australia). A clinical nurse specialist in an aged care setting who had used the collection as part of training commented that she believed, in part because of the use of this collection, "the staff are developing a better appreciation of the person behind dementia and not so focused on dementia itself" (survey response). "Classic" digital stories, with their emphasis on individual agency, the storyteller controlling their own narrative, and understanding that shared human experiences can allow emotional connections, clearly have potential to support training that is oriented towards person-centred care, even where the content of stories speaks more directly to the storytellers' personhood than experiences of care or of dementia itself.

Theorising practice: the emotional power of digital stories

Like Stenhouse and Tait, trainers using the digital stories for medical and health education who spoke to us stressed the emotional power of these materials to convey the experiences of people with dementia. One trainer described how she used one of the two digital stories included on the *Visual Stories* DVD which were made by people with dementia:

> I use David['s story]. I love it because he is not an actor. He's a real person with dementia and that's the message and he's speaking. ... He's the voice of people with advanced dementia. If we can take his words – he's still able bodied, he's still able to go out in public, he's able to be quite semi-independent and yet still he feels like he has no control over his life. He's scared, he becomes disorientated so he's feeling that in early stage ... If he's feeling that then, gosh, he's going to feel exactly the same things if not more when he's lost the voice to be able to articulate that.
>
>   (personal communication, dementia care trainer, Australia)

The feelings and anxieties David expresses in his story are seen as central to its value in training, in part because of the way people with dementia are often spoken of as if they are no longer present (Behuniak, 2011; Kitwood, 1997). Trainers suggested that digital stories helped listeners understand the feelings that may underpin the otherwise hard-to-understand actions of people with advanced dementia. In keeping with much work on the effectivity of digital storytelling, emotion was seen as a space of common ground between storyteller and listener by some teachers (Haigh & Hardy, 2011; Hardy & Sumner, 2014). Another trainer from Adelaide commented:

> residential care staff ... see a person when they come in at a certain level of dementia ... they forget this person was a ... fully functioning person at some stage but they don't see that. And when they see somebody like David or Cath who can articulate still and have got all these talents ... it sort of opens their eyes a bit ... A lot of people get quite teary.
>
>   (personal communication, dementia care trainer, Australia)

Hearing first-hand about the experience of people with dementia who are still able to articulate their experiences provokes an emotional response which is seen by this trainer as very powerful. Staff in dementia training centres pointed out that many people with advanced dementia rely on their emotions to function and so needed staff working with them to be able to communicate on that level.

Everyone we spoke to was aware of the challenges of staff opening themselves up to communication on an emotional level. As one Scottish trainer pointed out, nurses, for example, are often trained to keep up barriers to their emotions in order to protect themselves. Using emotion as a key route to communication with patients, she observed, was a challenge to such practices (personal communication). One manager in an Australian aged care centre whose role involved supporting students training to be allied health workers in work experience placements commented on the difficulties of using emotionally powerful digital stories in training. Given the lack of glamour of geriatrics as a specialism, the emotional power of these stories, especially when they are framed as tragic ones, is seen as potentially turning younger people away. "You need to use it well and debrief it and use it in a purposeful way ... you can actually do damage to staff ... why would you want to work in this area [if] it's going to break your heart?" (personal communication, aged care manager and trainer, Australia).

The emotional power of digital stories, and the access they might give to the experiences of people with dementia, might offer new insights for staff and open up new ways of communicating, but using them also required a new repertoire of professional skills in both trainers and the people they sought to train. The emotional challenges of exposure to powerful experiential narratives are by no means exclusive to dementia care training. Pip Hardy of Patient Voices powerfully describes digital storytelling facilitators as working "in the realm of suffering" (personal communication). As a consequence, Hardy and Sumner schedule regular clinical supervisions where they can talk through the emotional impact of what they have heard in the many storytelling workshops they facilitate.

These examples of the use of digital stories by people with dementia, their family members, and carers to teach nurses, medical students, and other health and social care workers have pointed towards the value of digital storytelling as an enduring alternative to the "hard gig" (personal communication) of a person with dementia speaking live to each new batch of trainees. Digital stories' realism, emotional power, and "fit" with the increasing emphasis on person-centred care in health (see for example, Nay et al., 2009; Nolan et al., 2004; Schwind et al., 2014) make them powerful training materials. However, the very emotional power of personal stories suggests that in understanding how such stories might best be used in educational settings, we need to think about emotional responses beyond empathetic responses.

Theorising listening: emotions and the pedagogy of discomfort

Frequently digital storytelling's power has been seen to rest in the empathetic connections it might encourage between listener and teller. However, the trainers we spoke to emphasised the much more complex range of emotional responses in training sessions, prompted by digital stories as well as other learning materials. Disinterest ("they don't want to be there"), defensiveness ("I've been working with people with dementia for 20 years – what can you tell me?"), and/or resistance to the idea that "challenging behaviour" might be attempts to communicate ("She can't truly be a nice person because she's presenting so horribly" (personal communication)) – were some of the reactions described in a focus group discussion with a group of Australian dementia care trainers. Kirk and colleagues have described their own responses to some of the stories they heard while collecting materials for the *Telling Stories* genomics education site as "professional shame" (Kirk et al., 2013, p. 523; see also Christiansen, 2011). This is a good way of describing some of the emotion articulated by health professionals in dementia training as they listen to stories by people with dementia and start to reframe their previous professional experiences. As one trainer commented:

> nurses are so motivated by caring, that's why you're in the profession, you don't think that something's gone to pieces because you did something wrong. ... if someone tells you you're missing the mark and you're not quite getting it right, that's confronting stuff.
>
> (personal communication, dementia care trainer, Australia)

Dealing with and helping people learn through such responses was seen as a key part of what dementia training was about. To be good at your job, as one Australian trainer said, "you can't stir it up and then not be able to take it anywhere or do anything with it. That's just destructive" (personal communication). In her philosophical exploration of listening, Susan Bickford notes that Aristotle viewed shame as a key moment in listening across difference. She observes that "someone who never feels the possibility of incompleteness will have difficulty genuinely hearing someone else" (Bickford, 1996, p. 151). The alterative, she suggests, citing Salkever's words, might be described as "the habitual disposition to worry that one's initial response to a situation might be wrong" (Salkever, cited in Bickford, 1996, p. 151). Yet to provoke productive listening such transformative emotions must be in the space between shame-lessness and "hopeless dread" (Bickford, 1996, p. 152). Dementia care trainers' descriptions of acknowledging and working with difficult emotions to prompt new kinds of listening evoke this account by Bickford of the preconditions of what she prefers to call "courageous listening" (pp. 152–153).

While empathy, prompted by emotional connection, is often seen as key to the power of digital storytelling, the accounts we heard of distress and distrust in dementia care training suggest, alongside such empathetic connections, a very different account of emotional listening for social change. Education scholar Megan Boler (1999) gives a very interesting description of her undergraduate literature students' responses to reading the famous semi-autobiographical graphic novel, *Maus* (Spiegelman, 1980–1991), which tells the story of the life and relationships of its author, the son of Holocaust survivors. Boler describes her concern when she suspects that her students, having read this powerful and affecting text, believe that they have a very complete understanding of the Holocaust. She dubs this response "passive empathy" – feeling one to have shared an experience because of your emotional connection to the storyteller. Boler's concern here was that, thanks to their sense of empathy, her students didn't seem to know what they didn't know. In the words of Eva Kittay (2009), they lacked "epistemological modesty".

Some of the trainers we spoke to offered similar accounts of the responses of people attending dementia care training. One trainer commented on the title "person centred care":

it's a lovely title but it's very easy to go, well "I'm a nice person and so that's what I do practise. I'm very much about the person, I'm very much about providing good care" ... unless people are challenged on it, they can look at it and go, "That's what I already do."

(Dementia care trainer, Australia)

Boler's critical account of this kind of empathy chimes with the work of other writers who have discussed the ways that the notion of empathy often elides differences between the feeling listener and the person with whom she empathises (e.g. Pedwell, 2012), via an assumption of shared "fellow feeling".

Along these lines. Boler argues for the value of another way of connecting to someone's life story – what she calls "testimonial listening". This kind of listening involves accepting:

a commitment to rethink her own assumptions, and to confront the internal obstacles encountered as one's own views are challenged ... What is at stake is not only the ability to empathise with the very distant other, but to recognise oneself as implicated in the social forces that create the climate of obstacles the other must confront.

(Boler, 1999 cited in Kelly, 2008, p. 18)

As many writers have pointed out, this acknowledgement of your own actions as an obstacle to others can be a deeply uncomfortable experience, especially perhaps to people whose professional self-conceptualisation is of being in the "helping professions" (McGloin, 2015; Ducey, 2007). Boler describes the kind of learning that might spring from this listening as "the pedagogy of discomfort".

Given the centrality of reflection as a strategy often turned to for professional learning, it's interesting to note that Schon, a key theorist of this process, viewed surprise or discomfort as prompts to this kind of reflection, where habit or "knowing-in-action" (Schon cited in Mann et al., 2009, p. 19) fail to explain an experience adequately. A widely reported outcome of reflection is also an increase in awareness of uncertainty (Mann et al., 2009, p. 614) – something that many people find uncomfortable. The notion of the "disorienting dilemma" in the work of Mezirow and other scholars of transformative learning similarly underlines the notion that discomfort and disorientation may prompt reflection and change (Mezirow, 1978).

The resisting responses to dementia care training suggest that these listeners had started to think through their status as, at least sometimes, obstacles rather than helpers for the people they worked with. The message we received from the dementia trainers we talked to, that dealing with strong emotions, including such resistance, was an essential and unavoidable part of the job, reinforces this conclusion. One dementia care trainer summarised the potential tensions for those working with people with dementia:

I always say to people, when you work in direct contact with people you have the most power to do harm and you can be criticized for that but you also have the most power to do good and to influence that person's wellbeing and to advocate for that person. ... You have to remember that you're part of the solution as well. ... The greater our understanding, the closer we can identify with that person as a fellow human being the more successful we are likely to be at that...

(personal communication, dementia care trainer, Scotland)

Listening pedagogies: pausable stories

So how can digital life stories be best used for professional education? Our conversations with trainers suggest they can be used in a range of ways, depending on their audiences, from junior doctors (who trainers the world over agreed were the most difficult audiences) to people retraining to work as domestic staff in aged care (personal communication). A shared view of those using digital stories to enhance care for people with dementia was that digital life stories were used not primarily to convey information, but rather to present the viewpoint of the person with dementia.

A number of the trainers we spoke to talked about a strategy for stories that would encourage professionals to imaginatively insert themselves in their role as professionals or decision makers into the narrative. While some trainers stressed the importance of "walking in the shoes" of people with dementia, others suggested that stories that are effective for learning not only prompt empathy with the experiences of the narrator, but encourage listeners to imagine their own responses as professionals who might have a role to play in the situation described by the narrator. As we have seen, listening to digital life stories, like dementia care education more broadly, can prompt discomfort and distress as well as empathy in listeners. These distressed professional listeners may be considering the possibility of their own complicity in the difficult circumstances of storytellers. Stories that allow trainees to imagine how they might act in the situations being described by storytellers are viewed by trainers as being potentially very valuable. This way of using digital life narratives might open up the possibility of health and social care workers considering how to be less of an obstacle to the people they work with. One trainer described such stories as "pausable stories" and a facilitator as "opaque" stories (personal communication):

sometimes we can just do a story and not put the outcome on the end of it and we will use that in the training to have the discussion with those present to see what their thoughts are, "how could you improve patient experience, patient pathway, what would you have done differently?" ... or just not play the outcomes, have that discussion, give every opportunity of giving their thoughts to us.

(personal communication, patient experience manager, Wales)

you can pause something and go "Right, so as a care worker if you were confronted with that, what would you be thinking and how would you respond?"

(personal communication, dementia trainer, Australia)

Stories that can be literally paused midway, or that prompt listeners to pause and reflect on the implications for professional practice, are seen as particularly productive by the people we spoke to. An experienced digital storytelling facilitator has suggested that stories can be more fruitful if they are more opaque because of the kind of reflection and listening that these less directive stories might invoke:

If you can leave it more opaque to a certain extent then people are less accusatory [rather than] "the hospital killed my brother and this is how". I'm not saying these things don't happen. But is it not better to say "This is what happened. This is what we saw happened and how it felt" … then the thinking around it and the reflection of that experience is easier to do and someone hasn't closed the door before you've even started on reflection.

(personal communication, digital storytelling facilitator, Wales)

The fact that the listener needs to reflect on and complete the story's "message" about professional practice is seen here as prompting reflection, where more accusatory narratives might prompt greater defensiveness.

This kind of interactive use of narratives drawn from life has been extended in Maggie Kirk's genomics team, by developing a role play exercise around the life experience story of an undiagnosed hereditary condition, its fatal implications for a family, and the ways in which various nursing and medical professionals might have intervened to change the outcome (personal communication). Such scenarios are familiar to educators and some students in health disciplines from influential problem-based learning approaches to professional education, but digital stories can be incorporated into such teaching occasions in a range of productive ways. Levett-Jones, Bowen, and Morris (2015) have drawn out the way this idea might work in online spaces by developing an interactive online virtual community whose inhabitants' experiences of health and care can be explored through digital stories embedded in specific physical and social locations throughout the site.

According to the accounts of the trainers and teachers who talked to us, such "pausable stories" encouraged listeners to connect stories to their own professional practice – to think about what they might have done in the situation being described, or to assess what could have been done differently. "Joining the dots" (personal communication) between life story narratives and the work of people listening to stories in training was seen as, in part, the role of trainers. Rather than simply encouraging empathy or fellow feeling, the activities which some trainers described building around these kinds of stories suggest something more like Boler's "testimonial witnessing" than the passive empathy of which she was so critical (Matthews, 2016). However, if some stories – more opaque or pausable, less "ranty" – are particularly "teachable" from the point of view of trainers, creating and using such stories is by no means ethically unproblematic.

Coaxing a teachable narrative

We want to think through here the implications of Sidonie Smith and Julia Watson's influential idea of a "coaxed narrative" for a pedagogy of listening. Smith and Watson (2001) argue that far from being simply an expression of self, various types of life narratives in the contemporary world are coaxed into being in particular social settings. Think of the curriculum vitae produced for a job application, the story that must be told at the unemployment office or on the form for disability benefits, the first meeting with a doctor or psychiatrist, the account of the defendant in a court hearing (Hall & Rossmanith, 2016; Matthews, 2007; Stanley, 2002). In all these different settings, to be successful, individuals need to "do good narrative" (Hall & Rossmanith, 2016). As Anna Poletti, citing Sidonie Smith and Julia Watson, put it: "individuals are called upon to produce an account of themselves which to be successful – that is to be intelligible to the intended audience – needs to achieve 'the right alignment of many kinds of evidence' into 'known scripts'" (cited in Poletti, 2011, p. 75).

While the idea of "coaxed narratives" might on the face of it suggest a distinction between "free" or "uncoerced" life stories and those that are wrenched out of people by powerful institutions, this idea has proven to be immensely productive precisely in fields where people are most interested in hearing – carefully hearing – the voices of marginalised people – in working-class and women's history for instance. Interestingly for our purposes, Anna Poletti has also used the notion of "coaxed narratives" to talk about the ways "specific" digital stories conform to particular themes and formats. Poletti does not set out to critique the stories that emerge from digital storytelling workshops but think carefully around what storytellers do and do not say, the constraints that both hedge storytellers in and make it possible for them to speak.

An interesting example of Smith and Watson's notion of a coaxed narrative emerged in a story told to us by the manager of a dementia training centre:

> We have a carer here that I've worked with for a long time … her husband has younger onset dementia … She's your typical Christian martyr. So she saves everyone else. … Her health is always bad, runs herself into the ground. Caring for her husband puts a real strain on her own life and capacity. And we did a radio interview with the ABC [public broadcaster Australian Broadcasting Corporation] where they … wanted to get to the hard stuff. She and I had just been talking about that, we were at an

event and the interviewer said "Have you got anyone?" [This carer] said "I'm very happy to share my story" … Well, when she got on the radio and I asked her how hard is it to be a carer. [She just said,] "Oh I love it, it's fine."

Our interviewee here is showing she is aware of the way life narratives are "coaxed". For instance she went on later in the interview to talk about the pressures on people to downplay their struggles by showing their awareness that "there's always someone worse off than me". Hinted at here are the powerful discourses of the selfless, even self-sacrificing wife and mother who does not complain about her lot in life. As Kathryn Knight (2015) has pointed out, this script is a difficult one to avoid for female carers, given the social opprobrium attached to expressing frustration or unhappiness with the caring role. Twentieth-century feminist history, with its emphasis on the way the difficulties of women's caring experiences are often concealed, makes it easier to see how this kind of story – of caring as an unmitigated pleasure – might be coaxed. Equally, second wave feminism's emphasis on the political value and importance of speaking out about personal experiences in the home gives us the sense of the political value of overcoming the narrative of the contented, self-sacrificing carer to speak about caring in other ways. The coaxed nature of this narrative is easily visible within this frame.

As pointed out by many scholars in disability studies, there's another, often contradictory, dimension to narratives of the difficulties of being a carer for a person with disability, one that's perhaps more difficult for non-disabled readers to see. Disability activists and scholars have pointed out the ways that narratives of disability as tragedy are one of the most widely accepted frames for talking about disability as an experience (Couser, 2003; Frank, 1995; Oliver, 1990; Sunderland, Kendall, & Catalano, 2009). Indeed, as Lorna Hallahan (2009) has pointed out, the kinds of narratives that are coaxed from people with a disability in bureaucratic encounters, like applications for funding or welfare support or in lobbying collectively for resources or changes to laws, are often such tragic stories, stories of "your worst day". In some respects, for the best of reasons, our respondent and the radio program were asking for just this kind of tragic story. Our interviewee saw such stories as an unfortunate necessity: "you also don't want to put real people in the position where you want them to tear their heart out in front of you … it's unfortunate, but without that you don't get the message across" (personal communication, dementia care trainer, Australia). Doing this ethically, she suggested is "around ensuring that the people that you work with are willing to bear themselves open, to really lay it all on the line on tape for public use, and that's a big ask" (personal communication). The emotional power of such stories, she suggested, is what makes them cut through in the wider domain of the media.

It might be argued that this story is an account of the real story of difficult caring being suppressed, rather than a coaxed narrative of a happy carer. This way of thinking enables us to maintain a distinction between the "true", unmediated story and the "false" story elicited via the mainstream media, and maintain the possibility of digital storytelling eliciting a "truer" if more painful account by removing media gatekeepers and conventions. However, despite the powerful tradition emphasising the importance of telling traumatic stories and the evidence all around us of such stories being actively suppressed by institutions like churches, governments, and media, it's important to remain alert to the ways in which traumatic and tragic stories are also often, in some respects, coaxed. Work on the ubiquity of life narratives has pointed out that such "coaxed" stories of selves are all-pervading in everyday life, and that our common-sense ways of thinking about ourselves and presenting ourselves are pervaded and framed within particular narratives in ways we may not always be fully aware of. As we will discuss in our account of the narratives offered in the consultation process for Australia's National Disability Insurance Scheme (NDIS) in Chapter six, often life stories are told within particular genres, using particular tropes, without little obvious prompting or encouragement. "Coaxed" narratives are not "coerced" narratives, but ones that people voluntarily feel it is possible and perhaps important to tell, in particular places, drawing on particular genres, in particular cultural and historical moments.

However, another example from our research points towards the ways that traumatic narratives can often be prompted in order to produce "teachable" moments. Ironically, this example emerges from a failure to produce a tragic narrative. In researching this chapter, we came across an example of a group of digital stories, in video form, that had been collected to document the experiences of gay, lesbian, and trans people and their journey with dementia. The stories were beautifully shot and absorbing stories, told to camera by people with dementia, about their experiences. One story, for example, narrated by a trans woman, includes a story of a very positive experience of coming out in military service. She offered to resign on announcing her transition, but her commanding officer wouldn't accept the resignation and sent her off to collect a women's uniform. Despite its charm and a very positive reception in the LGBTIQ community, this collection wasn't ultimately used as a teaching resource by the organisation that funded it.

The manager of the training organisation commented about the story:

> It's fantastic, if we were running a program I guess for people who were looking to transition and wanted to get that sense of, it's okay to be you. But the message we're trying to get out is it's a different message about the struggle and the discrimination faced by people and the marginalisation and the fear that they have in residential care … It doesn't really get to the point. What this particular project wanted was what is it like for someone like [the trans women in the video] [and particularly] the thought of going into residential care. And that is asking them to lay their soul bare and to think of the horrible things that may happen …

there's no way that we can inform a sector unless we have someone saying, "this is my experience". I met a wonderful intersex woman recently who talked about her issues with the care worker coming in, a very young Sudanese care worker coming in to shower her, and being confronted with the mixed genitalia ... the care worker just had to go, she ... didn't know what was going on ... they're the aha moments that I think are what needs to be translated.

(personal communication, dementia care trainer, Australia)

This story was, for the purposes of the organisation, then, in the wrong genre and about the wrong kinds of experiences. It was a story that fit well within the genre of a coming out narrative, and we could certainly think of this story as being "coaxed" in part through this celebratory genre. However, from the organisation's point of view, this collection of stories did not focus enough on discrimination and marginalisation to be useful as a teaching text, and to the best of our knowledge, it has not been used in training. This kind of outcome, where stories collected for training or other purposes are ultimately not circulated or used, is rarely described in published writing on digital storytelling, though we suspect it is not an uncommon outcome (for a rare exception of an account of such unpublished stories, see Gubrium, Hill, & Flicker, 2014).

In both of the examples we have given here, some staff we spoke to recognise the difficulties and hardships of telling traumatic stories, but insist that these are the kinds of stories that staff in the sector need to hear in order to improve things for people with dementia and their carers. We don't want to suggest that these trainers are wrong – there was a strong sense from many of the people we talked to in this field that stories of bad practice often offer good learning opportunities. However, we are troubled by the insistence that stories of trauma are key. Amy Hill (2008), working in a "classic" digital storytelling context, suggests that the specificities of particular stories are ways of moving beyond an oscillation between "narratives that are either problem-saturated and oppressive or relentlessly upbeat" (Hill , 2008, p. 49). The kinds of stories that Hill describes, and those solicited by Patient Voices in the *Dangling Conversations* project, are more like the kinds of stories that Lorna Hallahan calls for in valuing stories of "the disabled everyday". It may be that the challenges of producing teachable narrative articulated in the context we researched are avoided by more experienced story facilitators. However, the kind of conflict we have described here – between the desire of the storyteller to tell a particular story, and the sense by teachers and trainers of what might be a teachable story – is a real one, and not only in the context of digital storytelling in education but more broadly.

Coaxing a humanist narrative

Our conversations with dementia care trainers and teachers about the limits and value of digital storytelling as a resource for training suggest another way in which the "coaxed" narratives of digital storytelling might be problematic. As we discussed in Chapter two, Poletti's (2011) account of the underpinning values and assumptions of "classic" digital storytelling underscores the way a sense of shared human experiences and values underpins the philosophy of the movement. These values chime very well with the humanist understandings of subjectivity that underpin much dementia care training, particularly those of person-centred care that are central to dementia education settings (e.g. Brooker, 2003). As we have seen, reflective life storytelling by care workers is often used as a strategy for cultivating a sense of shared experience with people with dementia. For example, many texts used in training include exercises that encourage staff to write accounts of their own life, assemble a memory box, and reflect on what such exercises tell them about their clients' needs and histories. This shared philosophy is part of the reason for the pervasive use of life story in dementia care settings.

If empathetic responses based on a shared humanity are the ground on which much contemporary dementia education is founded, more recent scholarship around caring for people with dementia suggests some of the limitations of this approach. When it is evident that treating people with dementia as fellow human beings would be a huge advance on many current practices within institutionalised care, such perspectives seem hard to argue against.

However, recent accounts of caring for people with dementia draw out the importance of relationships in caring, and the way those relationships might shape subjectivity, in ways that extend the ideas of writers like Kitwood and begin to suggest the limits to a notion of shared human experiences as the only ground for better treatment of people with dementia. The notion of "malignant social psychology", and even more so, frameworks like relationship-centred care (Burke, 2014; Crichton & Koch, 2007; Keady & Jones, 2010), like the social model of disability, push towards a model of subjectivity as diverse, shifting, contextual, and relational, stretching humanist assumptions.

An emphasis on touch in approaches such as sensory therapy recognises different ways of communicating and the need to be present in ways that may be very different from most people's everyday interactions to provide comfort for people with advanced dementia. Anne Lidzey's (2004) poignant description of interacting with her mother, then in the final stages of dementia, through touch, breathing, and lip movements, in a way that evokes the interactions between a mother and a newborn, reminds us that we don't always ground a sense of humanness or worth in the ability to give an autobiographical account of the self. We acknowledge the necessary dependence of newborns on others – relationships with others are essential to their lives. We value the very young without expecting them to closely resemble those of us in mid-life or to have our range of skills and abilities, including our ability to talk about ourselves and our lives. Such approaches push against notions of similitude – a common life experience, a shared investment in individual biographical memory, a shared experience of uniqueness – as anchors for just and respectful treatment for people with dementia (Burke, 2014; Gibson, 2015). Taking seriously these human experiences that fall outside conventional understandings of what it means to be human – even as they are unexceptional – requires us to centre relationships and intersubjectivity as constituting ourselves. This stress on relationships and intersubjectivity is increasingly acknowledged in dementia care (Burke, 2014; Crichton & Koch, 2007; Keady & Jones, 2010).

Our conversations with dementia care trainers suggest that digital stories with their underpinning humanist assumptions, so valuable in asserting similitude and shared personhood, may not always be the most effective tool for underscoring the ways in which these relationships might unfold. A number of the scholars and dementia care educators we spoke to while researching this book expressed ambivalence about life story as a strategy for professional education in their field, despite its proliferation in various forms. The "tidiness" of the accounts of life story books by people with dementia seemed to some to underestimate the changes that might happen to people as they continue to live with dementia. Life story accounts were described as often done and put away, rather than forming part of the ongoing care, and evolving experiences, of people with dementia. As one trainer commented:

> life stories are dynamic. Life doesn't end when you go into the nursing home. So it should be added to as well and that's a challenge, getting people [to] go through that aspect … a person's tastes might change. People with dementia do learn new things and acquire new tastes, you know, they evolve.
>
> (personal communication, dementia care trainer, Scotland)

Digital storytelling with its focus on individual narratives may not capture the evolving lives of people with dementia or the role of carers in shaping people with dementia's experiences. This may make these narratives less valuable in dementia education that seeks to focus on relationships rather than other kinds of resources. Equally, as the examples discussed above suggest, the "malignant psychology" described by Kitwood that might shape the experiences of people with dementia in important ways may be hard to speak about in personal narratives.

Dementia education offers a kind of limit case of digital storytelling in professional education. Despite the ethical and practical challenges in collecting stories from people with dementia, the shared ground of "classic" digital storytelling and person-centred dementia education in the notion of universal human experiences as the basis for exchange, has made life-story telling a key strategy for education in this field. At the same time, the foregrounding of intersubjectivity in recent discussions of the experiences of dementia education, suggests some of the difficulties of relying on teaching tools that focus on individual stories outside of the contexts in which both individuals and their stories are shaped. As dementia care educators seek to turn their attention to the way care practices might profoundly shape the behaviour and experiences of people with dementia, they have frequently turned to other teaching tools in the quest to do this.

Navigating tensions between storytellers' aims and the "teachable" story

What can we draw from the case study of digital storytelling in dementia education for professional education more broadly? One important question that the case study of dementia education has broached is the potential conflict between the underpinning philosophy of the digital storytelling "movement" – giving the storyteller as much control as possible over the stories they tell – and the idea of digital storytelling as a tool that may be more or less fit for purpose. The conflicts between the different purposes of digital stories – the therapeutic narrative on the one hand and the teachable narrative, for instance – have been navigated in a number of different ways.

The ethical principles here might seem to be simple: just let storytellers tell the story they want to tell. But as storytelling facilitators pointed out to us, this naïve view of digital storytelling neglects the role of many elements that help to coax particular stories – the expertise and perspective of the facilitator themselves, the practices within workshops, and the genres of life storytelling that swirl around the narrator and are available to draw from: the coming-out story, for instance, the clinical history, or the tale of tragedy overcome.

One response to these difficulties has been simply to avoid using other people's life narratives for educational purposes, and reflect on your own story instead. The focus on reflection on one's own story has been one way of doing this, as we argued in the first part of this chapter. If one's own story is used as a teaching text, the narrative is still tethered to its teller and cannot be wrested from context. With the right kinds of prompts, narrators can make sense of the ways in which their own story might be framed and limited, which can be genuinely very useful for learning. Gubrium et al. (2014), for instance, have described how this process of reflecting on the ways in which storytellers' own accounts are shaped by prevailing metaphors, ideologies, and narratives might fit into activities taking place in the story circle (p. 1611). They describe a workshop in which young mothers were encouraged to reflect on the troublesome dimensions of ideas about teen mothers as lazy welfare recipients that emerged in some of their own stories. Similar reflection on representational issues might be prompted in the classroom.

A second approach, taken by Patient Voices and Rosie Stenhouse in the *Dangling Conversations* site, again draws heavily on reflection and metacognition by the listener. The "work" of reframing stories into learning opportunities is delegated to the student as listener. A few of these storytellers explicitly thematise their experiences of dementia, some in quite fragmentary ways, as the title of the project suggests. Others tell stories about their lives, and students, using the reflective questions offered by the project, need to think through what these stories might indirectly tell them about these individual people and their encounters with medical and social institutions, as well as with a medical condition.

Another strategy is to be quite selective about story collection, with a view to the kinds of stories that are likely to be useful in training contexts. Given the time taken to gather stories this was often seen as necessary from the point of view of staff trying to ration precious time (personal communication), but was also viewed as an ethical choice, as we will discuss in more detail in Chapter four. Ensuring that stories that were recorded would in fact be listened to was seen as very important by people adopting this perspective. Where stories might not be "teachable", those involved in gathering them might offer other possibilities for the teller – a formal complaints process, for example, or feedback in a written form into organisational decision making. As we discussed in Chapter two, Amy Hill of Silence Speaks argues that by framing both publicity and workshop prompts with care, it is possible for experienced story facilitators to be confident that stories that are collected can be used (see also Gubrium, Hill, & Flicker, 2014).

One facilitator, Lisa Heledd Jones of StoryWorks in Wales, navigated the tensions between teachable stories and the emphasis on storytellers' autonomy and control in participatory workshop traditions of digital storytelling by using a different word to describe stories led by organisational imperatives. She described commissioned projects in which organisations required a particular message to emerge from the collection of personal narratives as "films" rather than "digital stories" to flag up their different focus and the different locus of control of these stories.

Finally, some of the people we spoke to who had previously used digital storytelling for training were slowly moving away from drawing on life story. Showing students examples of bad practices was often seen as particularly helpful in getting them to think about their own activities. A number of the dementia trainers we spoke to in the organisation stressed the value of examples of bad practice, and noted that life storytelling may not always point out to practitioners the disparity between their own sense of being a good person with good intentions, and problematic care practices. One trainer noted the difficulty of getting staff who mean well to think through their own problematic processes. She imagines an internal monologue of someone in training:

> What you're wanting me to do is speak to people nicely and demonstrate relationship, person centred care. I know the buzz words and that's what you're meant to do and I'm a nice person. I already talk to people like that. ... I'm a good person and I'm motivated to provide good care.
> (personal communication, dementia care trainer, Australia)

She describes the shift in thinking she aims to make:

> When you start to paint a picture of who that person actually is and [what is] having an impact on their life – there's times where you just have silence. You can feel people going, 'Ah, yeah, I *do* do that.'
> (personal communication, dementia care trainer, Australia)

Many of the trainers we spoke to were alert to the ethical and practical difficulties of collecting narratives of bad practice, and some organisations had moved towards using fictional scenario-based audio-visual material in their training sessions to deal with this problem.

Take-aways for practitioners

- Deep reflection by storytellers doesn't necessarily produce deep reflection by listeners.
- Listening needs to be scaffolded – often the relevance of a particular story to a particular profession may need to be explicitly drawn out.
- The emotional power of life stories can make connections with listeners but can produce feelings of shame or resistance.
- An empathetic connection with the listener may allow listeners to ignore the role they may play in the difficult or "confusing situation" of the storyteller.
- Digital stories that allow professional listeners to consider what they should or could do in the situation being described can be engaging and useful for learning. Teachers and trainers need to be ready to deal and work with the emotional responses that may emerge from listening to these stories.
- There can be tensions between the needs of storytellers and the needs of organisations for "teachable" stories that need careful handling. Experienced facilitators have developed strategies for minimising these differences.
- In looking for a "teachable" story, think carefully about whether the story you have chosen repeats familiar and problematic narratives. Consider incorporating activities for listeners that involve reflecting on the familiar narrative types that individual stories may draw on.

Conclusions

Our examination of the ways that digital stories have – and have not – been used in education settings tells us important things about the challenges of using these resources, as well as our underlying preconceptions and values about learning from experiential narratives. As we have shown in this chapter, student-generated digital stories have been used widely in higher education to encourage students to reflect on their own knowledge and practice. Using storytelling this way fits neatly within a paradigm of learning that emphasises student agency and activity, as well as the metacognitive skills of reflection on one's own experience. This emphasis on using students' own digital stories has enabled teachers to avoid confronting some of the challenges of getting learners to listen to digital stories generated by others. As we have argued here, there are real opportunities for learning in such listening, particularly in areas like dementia care education, where retraining testimonial sensibilities and valuing individual voices are as important as sharing the content of stories. Listening to digital stories, then, can be very valuable for changing processes. However, we should not assume that there is necessarily a symmetry between reflective processes in the process of making stories and reflection in the process of listening to them.

References

Anderson, K. (2017, forthcoming). Digital storytelling as an avenue to deepen reflective social work practice. In Y. Nordkvelle, G. Jamissen, P. Hardy, & H. Pleasants (Eds.), *Digital Storytelling in Higher Education: International Perspectives.* Melbourne: Palgrave Macmillan

Barrett, H. (2006). Researching and evaluating digital storytelling as a deep learning tool. In C. Crawford, R. Carlsen, K. McFerrin, J. Price, R. Weber, & D. Willis (Eds.), *Proceedings of Society for Information Technology & Teacher Education International Conference* (pp. 647–654). Chesapeake, VA: AACE.

Behuniak, S. M. (2011). Oneself as another: Intersubjectivity and ethics in Alzheimer's illness narratives. *Ageing and Society, 31*(1), 70–92.

Benmayor, R. (2008). Digital storytelling as a signature pedagogy for the new humanities. *Arts and Humanities in Higher Education, 7*(2), 188–204. doi: 10.1177/1474022208088648

Bickford, S. (1996). *The Dissonance of Democracy: Listening, Conflict and Citizenship.* Ithaca, NY: Cornell University Press.

Boler, M. (1999). *Feeling Power: Emotions and Education.* Hove: Psychology Press.

Boud, D., Keogh, R., & Walker, D. (1985). *Reflection: Turning Experience into Learning.* London: Kogan.

Brooker, D. (2003). What is personcentred care in dementia? *Reviews in Clinical Gerontology, 13*(3), 215–222.

Brushwood Rose, C., & Low, B. (2014). Exploring the 'craftedness' of multimedia narratives: From creation to interpretation. *Visual Studies, 29*(1), 30–39.

Burgess, J. E. (2006). Hearing ordinary voices: Cultural studies, vernacular creativity and digital storytelling. *Continuum: Journal of Media and Cultural Studies, 20*(2), 201–214. doi: 10.1080/10304310600641737

Burke, L. (2014). Oneself as another: Intersubjectivity and ethics in Alzheimer's illness narratives. *Narrative Works, 4*(2), 28–47.

Burke, S. (2008). *Telling Stories, Understanding Real Life Genetics Educators' Perceptions of Relevance and Usefulness. Preliminary Report.* National Genetics Education and Development Centre.

Carel, H., & Kidd, I. (2014). Epistemic injustice in healthcare: A philosophical analysis. *Medicine, Health Care and Philosophy, 17*(4), 529–540.

Christiansen, A. (2011). Storytelling and professional learning: A phenomenographic study of students' experience of patient digital stories in nurse education. *Nurse Education Today, 31*(3), 289–293.

Conle, C. (2000). Narrative inquiry: Research tool and medium for professional development. *European Journal of Teacher Education, 23*(1), 49–63. doi: 10.1080/713667262

Coulson, D., & Harvey, M. (2012). Scaffolding student reflection for experience-based learning: A framework. *Teaching in Higher Education, 18*(4), 401–413.

Couser, G. T. (2003). *Vulnerable Subjects: Ethics and Life Writing*. Ithaca, NY: Cornell University Press.

Coward, M. (2011). Does the use of reflective models restrict critical thinking and therefore learning in nurse education? What have we done? *Nurse Education Today, 31*(8), 883–886.

Crichton, J., & Koch, T. (2007). Living with dementia: Curating self-identity. *Dementia, 6*(3), 365–381.

D'Alessandro, D. M., Lewis, T. E., & D'Alessandro, M. P. (2004). A pediatric digital storytelling system for third year medical students: The Virtual Pediatric Patients. *BMC Medical Education, 4*(10). doi: 10.1186/1472-6920-4-10

Davis, D. (2011). Intergenerational digital storytelling: A sustainable community initiative with inner-city residents. *Visual Communication, 10*(4), 528–540.

Ducey, A. (2007). More than a job: Meaning, affect and training health care workers. In P. Clough & J. Halley (Eds.), *The Affective Turn: Theorising the Social* (pp. 187–208). Durham, NC: Duke University Press.

Frank, A. W. (1995). *The Wounded Storyteller: Body, Illness and Ethics*. Chicago, IL: University of Chicago Press.

Fricker, M. (2003). Epistemic injustice and a role for virtue in the politics of knowing. *Metaphilosophy, 34*(1–2), 154–173.

Gibson, J. (2015). *(Not) the 'Right Kind' of Dementia Story: Re/Presenting Identities in Reality Theatre and Performance* (Doctoral dissertation). Sydney: Macquarie University.

Gidman, J. (2012). Listening to stories: Valuing knowledge from patient experience. *Nurse Education in Practice, 13*(3), 192–196.

Green, M., & Davies, K. (2009). RCN clinical leadership programme in action. *Nursing Management, 16*(7), 14–19.

Gridley, K. (2016). Life stories in dementia care: We all have a story and cannot be understood without it. *The Guardian*. Retrieved from https://www.theguardian.com/social-care-network/2016/apr/25/life-story-work-dementia-care

Gridley, K., Brooks, J., Birks, Y., Baxter, K., Cusworth, L., Allgar, V., & Parker, G. (2015). *Life Story Work in Dementia Care: Research Summary*. NIHR Health Services and Delivery Research. Retrieved from http://www.york.ac.uk/inst/spru/research/pdf/LifeStorySum.pdf

Gubrium, A., Hill, A., & Flicker, S. (2014). A situated practice of ethics for participatory visual and digital methods in public health research and practice: A focus on digital storytelling. *American Journal of Public Health, 104*(9), 1606–1614.

Haigh, C., & Hardy, P. (2011). Tell me a story – A conceptual exploration of storytelling in healthcare education. *Nurse Education Today, 31*(4), 408–411.

Hall, M., & Rossmanith, K. (2016). Imposed stories: Prisoner self-narratives in the criminal justice system. *International Journal of Crime, Justice and Social Democracy, 5*(1). Retrieved from https://www.crimejusticejournal.com/article/view/284

Hallahan, L. (2009, September). *Public testimony: Empowerment or humiliation?*The Story of the Story: Life Writing, Ethics and Therapy Conference. Adelaide: Flinders University.

Hardy, P. (2017, forthcoming). Physician know thyself: Using digital storytelling to promote reflection in medical education. In Y. Nordkvelle, G. Jamissen, P. Hardy, & H. Pleasants (Eds.), *Digital Storytelling in Higher Education: International Perspectives.* Melbourne: Palgrave Macmillan.

Hardy, P., & Sumner, T. (Eds.) (2014). *Cultivating Compassion: How Digital Storytelling is Transforming Healthcare.* Chichester: Kingsham Press.

Hessler, B., & Lambert, J. (2017, forthcoming). Threshold concepts of digital storytelling: Naming what we know about storywork. In Y. Nordkvelle, G. Jamissen, P. Hardy, & H. Pleasants (Eds.). *Digital Storytelling in Higher Education: International Perspectives.* Melbourne: Palgrave Macmillan.

Hill, A. L. (2008). Participatory media help Ugandan women who have experienced obstetric fistula tell their stories. Communication for Social Change Consortium. Retrieved from http://www.communicationforsocialchange.org/mazi-articles.php?id=417

Hull, G., & Katz, M. (2006). Crafting an agentive self: Case studies of digital storytelling. *Research in the Teaching of English, 41*(1), 43–81.

Jefferies, D., & Horsfall, D. (2013). Developing person-centred care through the use of autobiography. *International Practice Development Journal, 3*(1). Retrieved from http://www.fons.org/library/journal/volume3-issue1/article4

Jenkins, M., & Lonsdale, J. (2007, December). Evaluating the effectiveness of digital storytelling for student reflection (pp. 440–444). *ICT: Providing Choices for Learners and Learning Proceedings.* Ascilite Conference, Singapore. Retrieved from http://www.ascilite.org/conferences/singapore07/procs/jenkins.pdf

Kajder, S. (2004). Enter here: Personal narrative and digital storytelling. *English Journal, 93*(3), 64–68.

Keady, J., & Jones, L. (2010). Investigating the causes of behaviours that challenge in people with dementia. *Nursing Older People, 22*(9), 25–31.

Kearney, M. (2011). A learning design for student generated digital storytelling. *Learning, Media and Technology, 36*(2), 169–188. doi: 10.1080/17439884.2011.553623

Kelly, R. (2008). Testimony, witnessing and digital activism. *Southern Review, 40*(3), 7–22.

Kirk, M., Tonkin, E., Skirton, H., McDonald, K., Cope, B., & Morgan, R. (2013). Storytellers as partners in developing a genetics education resource for health professionals. *Nurse Education Today, 33*(5), 518–524.

Kittay, E. F. (2009). The personal is philosophical is political: A philosopher and mother of a cognitively disabled person sends notes from the battlefield. *Metaphilosophy, 40*(3–4), 606–626.

Kitwood, T. (1997). *Dementia Reconsidered: The Person Comes First.* Buckingham: Open University Press.

Knight, K. (2015). *Strange Country: Explorations through the Territory of Motherhood and Child Disability* (Doctoral dissertation). Sydney: Macquarie University.

Kocaman-Karoglu, A. (2016). Personal voices in higher education: A digital storytelling experience for pre-service teachers. *Education and Information Technologies, 21*(5), 1153–1168.

Lambert, J. (2009). The field of community arts. In J. Hartley & K. McWilliam (Eds.), *Story Circle: Digital Storytelling around the World* (pp. 79–90). Chichester: Wiley.

Large, S., Macleod, A., Kitson, A., & Cunningham, G. (2005). *A Multiple-Case Study Evaluation of the RCN Clinical Leadership Programme in England, Final Report to the Royal College of Nursing and the NHS*. Retrieved from https://www2.rcn.org.uk/__data/assets/pdf_file/0010/78643/002502.pdf

Levett-Jones, T., Bowen, L., & Morris, A. (2015). Enhancing nursing students' understanding of threshold concepts through the use of digital stories and a virtual community called 'Wiimali'. *Nurse Education in Practice, 15*(2), 91–96.

Lidzey, A. (2004). Coma work: A new approach to withdrawn states. *Journal of Dementia Care, 12*(3), 20–21.

Lowenthal, P. (2009). Digital storytelling: An emerging institutional technology? In J. Hartley & K. McWilliam (Eds.), *Story Circle: Digital Storytelling around the World* (pp. 252–259). Chichester: Wiley.

McDrury, J., & Alterio, M. G. (2002). *Learning through Storytelling: Using Reflection and Experience in Higher Education Contexts*. Palmerston North: Dunmore Press.

Mace, N., Coons, D. H., & Weaverdyck, S. E. (2005). *Teaching Dementia Care*. Baltimore, MD: The John Hopkins University Press.

McGloin, C. (2015). Listening to hear: Critical allies in Indigenous studies. *Australian Journal of Adult Learning, 55*(2), 265–280.

McKeown, J., Clarke, A., Ingleton, C., Ryan, T., & Repper, J. (2010). The use of life story work with people with dementia to enhance person-centred care. *International Journal of Older People Nursing, 5*(2), 148–158.

McWilliam, K. (2008). Australian digital storytelling as a "discursively ordered domain". In K. Lundby (Ed.), *Digital Storytelling, Mediatized Stories: Self-Representations in New Media* (pp. 145–160). New York: Peter Lang.

Mann, K., Gordon, J., & MacLeod, A. (2009). Reflection and reflective practice in health professions education: A systematic review. *Advances in Health Science Education, 14*(4), 595–621.

Matthews, N. (2007). Confessions to a new public: Video Nation shorts. *Media, Culture and Society, 29*(3), 435–448. doi: 10.1177/0163443707076184

Matthews, N. (2016). Learning to listen: Epistemic injustice and gothic film in dementia care training. *Feminist Media Studies, 16*(6), 1078–1092.

Meadows, D. (2003). Digital storytelling: Research-based practice in new media. *Visual Communication, 2*(2), 189–193.

Mezirow, J. (1978). Perspective transformation. *Adult Education, 28*(2), 100–110.

Mondal, A. (2016). *Protest/persuasion/performance: The ambiguities of liberal free speech theory*. Ethical Responsiveness: Listening and Reading across Difference Colloquium, University of Wollongong, March 18.

Nay, R., Bird, M., Edvardsson, D., Fleming, R., & Hill, K. (2009). Person-centred care. In *Older People: Issues and Innovations in Care* (p. 107). Chatsworth: Churchill Livingstone Elsevier.

Nolan, M. R., Davies, S., Brown, J., Keady, J., & Nolan, J. (2004). Beyond 'person-centred' care: A new vision for gerontological nursing. *Journal of Clinical Nursing, 13*(S1), 45–53.

O'Connor, D., Phinney, A., Smith, A., Small, J., Purves, B., Perry, J., Drance, E., Donnelly, M., Chadhury, H., & Beattie, L. (2007). Person hood in dementia care: Developing a research agenda for broadening the conversation. *Dementia, 6*(1), 121–142.

Oliver, M. (1990). *The Politics of Disablement: A Sociological Approach*. Melbourne: Palgrave Macmillan.

Pedwell, C. (2012). Affective (self-) transformations: Empathy, neoliberalism and international development. *Feminist Theory, 13*(2), 163–179.

Pfahl, N. L. & Wiessner, C. (2007). Creating new directions with story: Narrating life experience as story in community adult education contexts. *Adult Learning, 18*(3–4): 9–13. doi: 10.1177/104515950701800302

Pilgrim Projects (2016). *Patient Voices* [Website]. Retrieved from http://www.patient voices.org.uk/

Podkalicka, A. (2009). Young listening: An ethnography of YouthWorx Media's radio project. *Continuum: Journal of Media & Cultural Studies, 23*(4), 561–572.

Poletti, A. (2011). Coaxing an intimate public: Life narrative in digital storytelling. *Continuum: Journal of Media & Cultural Studies, 25*(1), 73–83. doi: 10.1080/10304312.2010.506672

Polk, E. (2010). Folk media meets digital technology for sustainable social change: A case study of the Center for Digital Storytelling. *Global Media Journal, 10*(17), n.p.

Pullman, D., Bethune, C., & Duke, P. (2005). Narrative means to humanistic ends. *Teaching and Learning in Medicine, 17*(3), 279–284.

Robin, B. (2006, March). The educational uses of digital storytelling. In C. Crawford (Ed.), *Proceedings of Society for Information Technology & Teacher Education International Conference* (pp. 709–716). Chesapeake, VA.

Robins, K., & Webster, F. (1999). *Times of the Techniculture. From the Information Society to the Virtual Life.* London: Routledge.

Rossiter, M., & Garcia, P. A. (2010). Digital storytelling: A new player on the narrative field. *New Directions for Adult and Continuing Education, 126*, 37–48. doi: 10.1002/ace.370

Royal College of Nursing (2004). *Clinical Leadership Toolkit.* London: Royal College of Nursing.

Sadik, A. (2008). Digital storytelling: A meaningful technology-integrated approach for engaged student learning. *Educational Technology Research and Development, 56*(4), 487–506.

Sandars, J., & Murray, C. (2009). Digital storytelling for reflection in undergraduate medical education: A pilot study. *Education for Primary Care, 20*(6), 441–444.

Schwind, J. K., Lindsay, G. M., Coffey, S., Morrison, D., & Mildon, B. (2014). Opening the black-box of person-centred care: An arts-informed narrative inquiry into mental health education and practice. *Nurse Education Today, 34*(8), 1167–1171.

Sheard, D. (2008). *Growing: Training that Works in Dementia Care.* Feelings matter most series. Brighton: Alzheimer's Society.

Smeda, N., Dakich, E., & Sharda, N. (2014). The effectiveness of digital storytelling in the classrooms: A comprehensive study. *Smart Learning Environments, 1*(6), n.p. doi: 10.1186/s40561-40014-0006-0003

Smith, S., & Watson, J. (2001). *Reading Autobiography: A Guide for Interpreting Life Narratives.* Minneapolis: University of Minnesota Press.

Spiegelman, A. (1980–1991). *Maus.* New York: Pantheon Books.

Stanley, L. (2002). From 'self-made women' to 'women's made-selves': Audit selves, simulation and surveillance in the rise of the public woman. In T. Cosslett, C. Lury, & P. Summerfield (Eds.), *Feminism and Autobiography: Text, Theories, Methods* (pp. 40–60). London: Routledge.

Stenhouse, R. (n.d.). *Dangling Conversations. A Collection of Digital Stories Made by People with Early Stage Dementia.* Albertay University. Retrieved from https://app lications.abertay.ac.uk/external/Schools/SHS/DanglingConversations/

Stenhouse, R., & Tait, J. (2014). *Dangling conversations* – digital storytelling with people with early stage dementia. In P. Hardy & T. Sumner (Eds.), *Cultivating Compassion: How Digital Storytelling is Transforming Healthcare*. Chichester: Kingsham Press.

Stenhouse, R., Tait, J., Hardy, P., & Sumner, T. (2013). *Dangling conversations*: Reflections on the process of creating digital stories during a workshop with people with early-stage dementia. *Journal of Psychiatric and Mental Health Nursing, 20*(2), 134–141.

Sunderland, N., Kendall, E., & Catalano, T. (2009). Missing discourses: Concepts of joy and happiness in disability. *Disability and Society, 24*(6), 703–714. doi: 10.1080/09687590903160175

Thompson-Long, B., & Hall, T. (2017, forthcoming). Digital storytelling and design-based research: Designing for deeper reflection in post-primary teacher education. In Y. Nordkvelle, G. Jamissen, P. Hardy, & H. Pleasants (Eds.), *Digital Storytelling in Higher Education: International Perspectives*. Melbourne: Palgrave Macmillan.

University of Stirling (2012). *Best Practice in Dementia Care: A Six Part Self-Study Course for Domiciliary Staff*. Stirling: The Dementia Services Development Centre.

Walsh, D. (2006). *Dementia Care Training Manual for Staff: Working in Nursing and Residential Settings*. JKP Resource Materials.London: Jessica Kingsley.

Wexler, L., Eglinton, K., & Gubrium, A. (2014). Using digital stories to understand the lives of Alaska Native young people. *Youth & Society, 46*(4), 478–504.

4 Listening for service improvement in primary and acute health care settings

In this chapter, we move beyond the context of professional education to explore the impact of digital stories in primary and acute health care settings. Over the last few decades, the public have come to expect people who manage and deliver health services to listen to service user voices, but it is still not clear whether this practice is creating better patient outcomes. We aim to shed some light on this topic, by unpacking some of the ways that digital storytelling has been used to enhance primary and acute health care, and theorising practices of listening to personal stories within the context of health care services. We will do this by examining a number of case studies of digital storytelling based in the United Kingdom (UK), particularly the 1000 Lives Plus project in Wales (NHS Wales, n.d.) and Pip Hardy and Tony Sumner's Patient Voices (Pilgrim Projects, 2016). These case studies draw on documents and stories, as well as conversations with people who have attempted to incorporate patient stories within health care decision-making processes.

The rise of the service user voice in the British National Health Service

Both of the case studies in this chapter are based in Britain, so we will begin this chapter with a discussion of the context of the political and public shifts that have brought the question of patient stories and experiences to the fore within the British National Health Service (NHS). While the UK has a distinctive system of socialised medicine as a public service, public and service user involvement in the governance of health services, and patient choice and control over their treatment, have been noted in a range of international contexts (Armstrong, Herbert, Aveling, Dixon-Woods, & Martin, 2013; Hardy & Sumner, 2014; Kvarnstrom, 2011; Li, Abelson, Giacomini, & Contandriopoulos, 2015; Renedo, Marston, Spyridonidis, & Barlow; 2015; Topol, 2015; Tovey, Atkin, & Milewa, 2001).

Some popular writers, such as Eric Topol in his 2015 account of "patient power", *The Patient Will See You Now*, have viewed the rise of the patient as co-producer of medical knowledge as being driven by technology. We think it's more complex than that. The rise of the service user voice in Britain's NHS offers a fascinating example of the way that pressures from very different groups and political perspectives can converge on a particular set of languages that work in very divergent vocabularies. The diverse forces pressing for public and patient participation in the provision of health services include neoliberal political traditions with their distrust of state-run services and emphasis on patient choice, the critiques of medical paternalism from feminism and the disability movement, and calls for a more responsive and diverse health service from under-serviced groups (Tovey et al., 2001). Graham Martin (2008) argues that the imperatives behind an emphasis on patient and public involvement in health services across the political spectrum throughout the Western world spring from two distinguishable but overlapping perspectives: a sense of democratic deficit in the way that policies and institutions have played out, and a desire to reorganise or "reform" welfare systems to respond to perceived changes in contemporary societies.

The heightened political prominence of the service user's voice can be also be connected to the disability movement. Disability activist and scholar critiques of medical paternalism, and calls for "nothing about us without us", have been important precursors to the current rhetorical emphasis on patient voice. Earlier liberation movements, such as the anti-psychiatry movement and feminist push for women's health from the 1960s, had critiqued centralised, bio-medical, and technologised approaches to health. These movements called for the health service user to play a key role in decision making around their own health. Such calls were often embedded within alternative paradigms of health – holistic, political, socio-cultural understandings that demanded shifts in the hierarchies of expertise within medicine, and changes to the kind of knowledge valued as sources of health information.

These broader claims about inadequacies in the health system have been reinforced over the last twenty years by the outcomes of a number of inquiries into clinical failures. Robert Francis' (2013) report into preventable deaths under the care of the Mid-Staffordshire Foundation Health Trust, for example, which prompted widespread re-examination of practices in the UK's NHS, framed some of the organisational problems as a failure to adequately listen to patients and staff (Spencer, Puntoni, & Matthias, 2015). Attending to patient voices has been seen as a remedy for these problems. The Kennedy Inquiry in 2001, for instance, said that "patients must be treated as partners by health professionals and treated as 'equals with different expertise'" (Kennedy, 2001 cited in O'Neill, 2014, p. 68). More recently, the Berwick Inquiry, which focused on improving patient safety in Britain, proposed a principle that the NHS should systematically and continuously "engage, empower and hear" patients and carers (National Advisory Group on the Safety of Patients in England, 2013, p. 43).

These voices were joined by supporters of neoliberal approaches to public policy, particularly those viewing state-managed and state-funded public health as inevitably inefficient and paternalistic. While feminists, disability activists, and other community representatives often sought to continue or extend socialised systems of managing health, right-wing critics of the NHS saw privatisation and more control over the organisation of health by individual practitioners and local health trusts as a solution to state control (Martin, 2008; Tovey et al., 2001). A view of health as not so much a public service but a consumer good, to be chosen by individuals with access to information and purchasing power from an array of providers, was put forward by conservatives as a rival model to state provision of services. It has been argued that at various times – for instance, in the late 1990s and early 2000s in the UK – this consumer paradigm was supplemented by more participatory conceptions of public and patient involvement in health (Martin, 2008; Stewart, 2011). While Stephen Harrison and Maggie Mort have pointed out that "being in favour of better public consultation or more user involvement is rather like being against sin; at a rhetorical level, it is hard to find disagreement" (Harrison & Mort, 1998, p. 66), the complexity of divergent aims and motives undergirding patient and public involvement in the governance of health has shaped the responses – and sometimes the resistance of health professionals – to such moves (Davies, Powell, & Rushmer, 2007, p. 128).

In describing the way digital storytelling has been used in organisational settings, we move beyond simple binaries to understand power plays around storytelling in health service improvement. Clearly people working within the health service, particularly medical and nursing staff, have power in relation to the people they care for. However, at a time when British junior doctors are striking to resist new contracts that would increase their hours and reduce their rate of pay, a more nuanced account of power in the health service that considers gendered, racialised, and classed identities, alongside the power of biomedicine and expertise, is needed (see for example, Dyer, McDowell, & Banitzky, 2008). When our informants speak of the health service as "massively dysfunctional", they're often talking not just of the arrogance and distance of medical staff or the pre-eminence of biomedical and clinical models of knowledge, but of the complex consequences of funding cuts and changes to work practices, layered over older problems. This complexity suggests the need for caution about simple or utopian accounts of the power and politics of digital storytelling in health care settings.

Case study: Institutionalised listening

So how have life stories been used with the intention of improving services in the British NHS? In exploring this question through this chapter we have used documentary and multimedia evidence available in the public sphere in addition to documents provided by 1000 Lives Plus and Pilgrim Projects. These case studies were supplemented by in-depth interviews conducted between 2014 and 2016. Formal interviews were conducted under an approved ethics protocol via Macquarie University. Stakeholders in this case study have only been identified based on their express request to be so.

Our research into the use of multimedia narratives of personal experience for service improvement in health has uncovered a range of uses of digital stories. As a number of our respondents have emphasised, there has been increasing buy-in to the idea of collecting and using patient stories as part of the evaluation of patient experience in Wales, as elsewhere in the UK, at the highest levels of management. As one respondent commented, "I think the steer from the top sends a very big message down to the staff right down from middle management down to lower management and if you haven't got that right, then actually it's always a bit of a carte blanche for the staff to say, 'We don't have to do that.'" Robert et al.'s (2011) report, entitled *What Matters to Patients?* (commissioned by the English NHS), featured as its first recommendation the need to "recognise and maximise the value of patient stories" (p. 28). This report noted that most surveyed NHS organisations were committed to collecting patient stories. Sarah Puntoni, who played a key role as Healthcare Improvement Lead Officer for the Welsh NHS's 1000 Lives Plus project, commented, "there is an appreciation at all levels of the organisation of stories. To hear stories when you go to meetings and events now is not unusual. It is fairly normal these days" (personal communication).

Pip Hardy and Tony Sumner of Pilgrim Projects have possibly the longest and best-documented record of using digital storytelling in a sustained and targeted way for health service improvement, having started using digital stories while considering practices around clinical governance. Their recent edited collection, *Cultivating Compassion*, which documents the history, philosophy, and impact of their Patient Voices endeavour, describes more than 100 projects using digital storytelling in the health arena, primarily in the UK (Hardy & Sumner, 2014). Outside the use of stories in professional education discussed in Chapter two, the most commonly reported use of stories is in within board meetings, as we will discuss in more detail in the case study below. Stories are also widely used in in-service training – in the Welsh NHS recorded stories have been used in corporate training by patient experience managers for those new to the NHS, "preceptor" training for new nurses, and training around patient experience for medical students and junior doctors. However, stories are also used for public dissemination of research findings and enquiries (see for example, Stanton, 2014; Taylor & Hardy, 2014), as part of evaluation processes (Hardy & Sumner, 2014), as tools for prompting change in governance processes (Hardy & Sumner, 2014), to debrief difficulties encountered by teams (Stabler, 2014), and as part of interview processes for senior appointments (Haigh, Cahoon, & Sumner, 2014).

Co-design is another approach to the use of digital stories (see for example, O'Neill, 2014). In a rich account of a large-scale use of storytelling for co-design of health services, Locock and colleagues (2014) describe an accelerated experience-based co-design approach to service improvement, drawing on the extensive collections of over 3,000 recorded interviews from the public site *HealthTalkOnline*. In this research project, narratives from the *HealthTalkOnline* collection were used as a trigger for analysis by groups of patients and families, and with staff – generating areas and strategies for improvement. The narratives were not recorded for this particular research project, but were recorded elsewhere in the country. Locock and colleagues (2014) emphasised the importance of the conversation between health service provider and patients as a powerful motive for reflection. While the "trigger" stories weren't connected to the patients and communities involved in the co-design process, Locock and colleagues viewed the ongoing presence of patient groups as helping to ensure that action ensues from the identification of issues that both storytelling and the discussion of stories with professionals enable (Locock et al., 2014).

As we have emphasised throughout this book, the mediation of a story and its movement from its teller to new spaces are both exciting and worrying to many invested in participatory processes for creating such stories. Practitioners that we spoke to were highly engaged with the ethical implications of moving stories away from their tellers. Maximising the use of digital stories was one of the ethical principles that was most clearly articulated to us. The 1000 Lives Plus project in Wales, for example, advocates a range of uses for digital stories for education, inspiration, and service enhancement, and consequently offers a useful instance to think through these questions. As documented in Chapter three, the use of patient stories in the Royal College of Nursing's Clinical Leadership program had an influence on the way digital stories were used for service improvement in the 1000 Lives Plus project in the Welsh NHS. Protocols in the Clinical Leadership program suggested that stories should be destroyed after being used for mind mapping and service enhancement.

Yet, Sarah Puntoni of the 1000 Lives Plus project viewed failing to reuse stories as, in essence, unethical. Puntoni commented that, "the majority of people who give the story ... because they want to be heard ..., especially if there's a negative element to it. They want the organisation and the individual to learn from it and for it not to happen again." Consequently, she observed that "in my experience people are usually very happy for people to have stories shared for the purposes of improvement" (personal communication). Anna Tee and Jonathon Gray's guidance from 1000 Lives Plus on using stories (Tee & Gray, 2012) hence emphasises the importance of ensuring that consent is sought for a range of different uses.

The 1000 Plus Lives project guidelines proposed that patient stories could be used for the following purposes: for learning to improve the service and educate new staff; for inspiration such as "motivational reminders to frontline staff of why they do what they do"; and for the media in order to "change a public mindset", "endorse good work", and "draw attention to flaws in the system and to validate 1000 Lives plus" (Tee & Gray, 2012, p. 21). The guidelines note the potential value of stories for research, but this is seen as a process with quite distinct and separate processes, notably the requirement for formal ethics approval, and is not seen as central to the use of stories in the organisation.

Using patient stories in formal meetings

Patient stories, in a range of forms, have become a regular feature of formal meetings, such as public boards, quality committees, learning panels, and patient experience or safety panels, across the UK (Haigh et al., 2014; Robert et al., 2011; Taylor & Hardy, 2014). Sometimes these stories are presented in person by the service user themselves. More commonly, edited excerpts of audio or video recording, "specific" digital stories, or text-based stories are brought into the meeting, often included at its beginning as a way of "setting the tone". What is the purpose of using patient stories in formal meetings, such as public board meetings? Robert et al.'s (2011) *What Matters to Patients?* report commented on the rationale for the existing use of patient stories in this way:

> Many NHS boards have created opportunities to listen to patients' stories, typically focusing on complaints and adverse incidents more regularly than the more day-to-day or even the better experiences. Stories provide a more vivid and immediate medium for communicating experiences than formal reports using graphs and data; they keep staff sensitive to patients' experiences, create more readily a sense of ownership and motivate staff to find solutions to problems. In most of the sites, stories were the only method in use for capturing issues to do with continuity of care and transitions between sectors.
>
> (Robert et al., 2011, p. 21)

Given the high priority afforded to patient experiences of transitions in care in the NHS Constitution, the fact that patient stories are seen in this report as a key way of mapping patient experiences highlights their value in this political moment, despite the mismatch between such qualitative inputs, and the types of data on clinical outcomes and safety that have historically been valued. Indeed, the Francis report called for greater attention to be "paid to the narrative contained in, for instance, complaints data, as well as to the numbers" (Francis, 2013, p. 90).

Staff involved in collecting stories around patient experience saw the holistic nature of stories as key to their effectiveness in boards. Sarah Puntoni commented:

> The whole idea at board level at least is to get them to realise that the decision they make has an impact for people's lives. So in some cases it might be about getting them to understand something that is quite a complex issue, but in a majority of cases it's just to get them to make that connection, to really understand what people are feeling.
>
> (personal communication)

Including stories in the most significant formal meetings of Health Trusts is also a way of indicating the importance placed on patient experience. Haigh et al. (2014) argue that including stories in boards "focus[es] the attention of the board members on the reasons for their meeting (to run a Trust that provides care for service users) and ... place[s] the voice of the patient at the heart of the decision making process" (p. 90). A clear signal from organisational leaders that the experience of patients is of central importance was seen as key by the patient experience managers we spoke to. One manager in the NHS involved with collecting patient stories commented:

> I think definitely if we're going to take service user experience seriously there has to be that very strong steer from the top to say, "this is what we're doing, these are the reasons why, there are great benefits to this", and that has to be passed down through the ranks really.
>
> (personal communication, NHS manager)

Sometimes patient stories are presented in person by service users themselves or by their families, rather than being recorded and edited. Having service users present at board meetings was widely viewed as the most powerful way of incorporating the patient voice. One manager commented, "in my experience, [it is] far better to have the person in the room, rather than have the virtual person because the actual person has a far greater impact than any other format you're likely to bring" (personal communication, NHS manager). Yet, having a storyteller come into a board meeting was seen as requiring careful preparation and negotiation of the needs and exposure of the storyteller, in line with publicly accessible case studies and guides from the 1000 Lives Plus project (Heywood, Puntoni, & Spencer, 2012).

Patient experience managers and others involved in negotiating the presence of a storyteller at a board noted that the formal style of board meetings meant that they were not always a welcoming environment for patients talking about their own experiences. Armstrong et al.'s (2013) work on patient and public involvement in the NHS noted that in formal settings such as boards, patient "contributions may be limited by their lack of familiarity with the system's language and norms and by power differentials" (p. e37). Those arranging for service users to attend boards and tell their stories were also concerned at the conflict between a respectful approach to the storyteller – allowing them to expand on their experiences for as long as they would like – and the inevitable concern for time in public board meetings. As one respondent commented, "For me, if you're going to bring someone into a meeting, whether they go on for an hour or ten days, you must listen to them because you've asked them to come to that meeting" (personal communication, NHS manager, Wales). In the words of another patient experience manager, using recorded stories was seen as the NHS staff involved in collecting stories "managing that time pressure" (personal communication, patient experience manager, Wales). Another interviewee commented, "We tend to not give them the time and the space that I think is respectful. … I think it's really rude to say to somebody, 'You've had this really bad experience and you've come to [the] board but you've only got five minutes to talk about [it]'" (personal communication, patient experience manager, Wales).

While those involved in collecting stories within the NHS viewed individuals' experiences as an extremely important source of information about quality of care, patient experience managers reported that some board members viewed individual stories as failing to be representative: a concern drawn in part from more familiar ways of approaching problem analysis in a scientific mode. Patient experience manager, Anna Tee, commented:

> I've seen it where they've started on telling their own story, people will do the "well, but that's just you" type thing and I find people will dismiss it. And the patient will get annoyed and upset because they feel that their experience is being belittled but the service will expect people to be a representative.
>
> (personal communication, patient experience manager, Wales)

As Armstrong and colleagues (2013) note, the personal qualities that mean patients are willing to participate in formal governance procedures can fuel claims that such patients are not representative of their peers (see also Renedo et al., 2015). This question of representativeness has also been foregrounded in both Labour and Conservative policy documents around patient involvement in health (Martin, McKee, & Dixon-Woods, 2015).

Emotive and negative stories

Some project facilitators indicated that the high level of emotion in stories that might be told "live" could be problematic. The digital storytelling facilitators and patient experience managers we spoke to often commented that "ranty" stories were less effective in prompting change than more "balanced" or emotionally ambiguous stories. Tony Sumner from Patient Voices, for example, noted "something that's just a 12 minute rant at the audience, people would turn off after 12 seconds" (personal communication, digital storytelling facilitator, England). A patient experience manager wanted to avoid the aggression that might emerge from a storyteller seeking "to see the whites of their eyes!" (personal communication) when her story was told in a public board. Some patient experience managers' preference for recorded stories that "manage" the emotional tone of narratives would be seen as politically problematic by many self-advocates. The "management" of raw emotion in these narratives, and the shaping of their affective power, might be seen as instances of professionals and organisations refusing to listen or limiting their listening to certain conditions. Patient experience managers, in contrast, presented the process of hearing out the service user's full story and then condensing it into a recorded narrative as a way of giving storytellers space to express their anger and frustration while at the same time shaping the story in ways that would be "listenable" by the institution.

Robert and colleagues' (2011) *What Matters to Patients?* report indicated that the use of stories in boards often focuses on "adverse" incidents. The more recent Berwick Report also acknowledged limitations of this focus on "blame as a tool" (National Advisory Group on the Safety of Patients in England, 2013, p. 10). Some patient experience managers in our study were also very critical of folding patient stories into the complaints process. Complaints were investigated and adjudicated by the health service, a process which one patient experience manager saw as fundamentally at odds with the underpinning philosophy of patient stories as representing the perspective of the storyteller. She commented:

> We're very used to complaints processes where we investigate and we uphold or not, a complaint. My view is, and I've said this to senior management – how arrogant are we! How arrogant are we that we say "no that didn't happen". Of course it happened in that person's understanding! ... We investigate them and we send these awful letters back to people saying "This is basically what happened in our opinion". If it's different from what happened in their opinion then we're kind of saying, I think the unsaid implication is, "you're a liar". If somebody's taken the effort to write a complaint then we should respect that and say "thank you very much for that information".
>
> (personal communication, patient experience manager, Wales)

Collapsing the distinction between stories and complaints is seen as reasserting a hierarchy of knowledge between professionals and patients, even at the moment where that hierarchy might be seen to be breaking down.

Responses to stories

The ways in which stories might be used in formal meetings to enhance service delivery and outcomes were mapped out in a description of the way an audio story was used in a formal panel designed to feed patient experience into a range of disparate services in a geographically diverse health trust. The manager charged with bringing stories to the panel described the process in this way:

> That was a story that was developed verbally as in an audio clip but what we then did was, I developed a template, just because it was the one we did though the panel ... we looked at all the positives and we looked at the negative areas of somebody's experience through that service and then we pulled out [issues ... I]t was funny as I'm not in that service area. I'm across them but I'm not in the day to day running of that so I'm detached almost ... all the things that I pulled out she also pulled out, which was quite reassuring and good. And then what she did was she took it back to her programme board, and her programme board which is like an internal meeting that they have with staff and then they discussed some of those areas about how they could be improved and so on, and then

because there were some of those areas that were outside the scope of [the health trust], she took them into those meetings ... where she thought that people needed to know. So she shared that information.

(personal communication, NHS manager, Wales)

Our interviewee admitted that this was an example of good practice that wasn't always evident in the use of digital stories, a point also noted in Robert and colleagues' *What Matters to Patients?* report:

Strikingly, over 95% of the time, the minuted action point on patient experience is to note the report and take no further action. Examples where patient experience data is used to spark debate and action were rare, as were examples of non-executive directors challenging performance.

(Robert et al., 2011, p. 16)

The Manchester Mental Health and Social Care Trust offer a useful instance of the ways in which stories might be framed in boards to enhance the chance of outcomes emerging from their use. Carol Haigh, Patrick Cahoon, and Tony Sumner (Haigh et al., 2014) observed that in Manchester, "when the stories are shown to the Board, they are tasked with articulating the top three actions that will be taken to assure themselves that issues described in the stories are less likely to happen in future" (p. 90). This process is reflected in the approach taken by Patient Voices within their celebratory screening (Hardy & Sumner, 2014). Listeners are given post-it notes and asked to jot down the way a story made them feel, what it made them think, and what they might do in response.

Tying featured patient stories into key meeting agenda items was seen as a useful strategy by a number of the patient experience managers we spoke to. Manchester Mental Health and Social Care Trust takes this notion of linking agenda items, personal stories, and opportunities to draw out any implica-tions a step further. Tony Sumner of Patient Voices describes the strategy used in Manchester:

[The Trust] for example, uses – takes basically one story from a workshop every month back to its board [... T]heir engagement manager picks a story for the month. Gets the storyteller who told the story in. They sit down together, look at the themes in the story, they write a shared position paper on the organisation's position with regard to whatever those things are. Whether they are poor housing for people with mental health service issues, drug concordance, crime, that sort of stuff. Then they both, together, take that paper back and present it to the board as a way of illuminating – not that patient, that service user's experiences. But using the service user's experiences as a lens through which to view the behaviour of the organisation itself. So that's one very powerful way of doing it.

(personal communication, digital storytelling facilitator)

This approach addresses concerns about patient voice representativeness as well as building an ongoing relationship with the storyteller that reflects the participatory ethic of "classic" digital storytelling, and echoes the co-design approach discussed by Locock and colleagues (2014).

Perhaps in response to the remarks of the Robert report, increasingly there is a visible effort by services drawing on patient stories to document the ways they have been used and listened to. For example, the most recent collection of digital stories on the Welsh Ambulance Service site are embedded as links within a description of the ways in which the story was shared as part of the Ambulance Service's Board meeting or Quality, Patient Experience and Safety Committee. A number of these descriptions included changes to practice being considered or evaluated as a consequence of listening to the story. Several older digital stories in a separate part of the site also include narratives of "what happened next" – for instance, further training for paramedics in ways of supporting people with laryngectomies in the wake of the story *Concern for Dad*, a "specific" digital story by a daughter who was offered little support by ambulance staff when her father's breathing tube slipped out in a coughing fit.

Case study: Reshaping epistemological communities in the Welsh NHS

Drawing on the case studies in Chapters two and three, we argue that there is a kind of dance or negotiation between tellers and listeners, hosts, caretakers, and brokers when stories of personal experience are circulated and used. This negotiation relates to professional norms and beliefs around which stories are safe or good to tell, and which stories are listenable for particular people in particular institutional locations. Battles over the way that different kinds of stories are able to be heard emerged in our discussion of digital storytelling in training in Chapter two. For instance, in one digital storytelling project funded by government, a storyteller's choice of images of dolphins leaping and flowers blooming to illustrate a story about the experience of dementia was initially seen by funding bodies as inappropriately "arty" to be an effective form of communication (personal communication, dementia care trainer, Australia). This theme emerged again as we talked to facilitators and patient experience managers in the Welsh NHS. Using digital stories in a strategic or instrumental way, posed the challenge of how (or if) the stories that health service users wanted to tell contributed to the health service changes that storytellers wanted to see. A key part of this process was making stories "listenable" to the organisation and professionals within it – a process that, in the wider context of the NHS, Karen Taylor and Pip Hardy have called an "evidence revolution" (Taylor & Hardy, 2014, p. 75).

Projects such as 1000 Lives Plus are actively seeking to reshape Welsh service providers' understanding of what constitutes important information about health. Practitioners working in this area – neither marginalised nor fully empowered, often working as non-clinical staff in clinical contexts, stressing the value of narratives and experience as data against biomedical emphasis on measurement of clinical outcomes in quantitative forms – are navigating a field of power and hierarchies of evidence, in which constant negotiations about what is listenable, teachable – what works – take place.

In Chapter three, we used Miranda Fricker's (2003) notion of testimonial sensibility to consider the ways in which digital storytelling was used by dementia care educators to try to reshape professional carers' interpretations of the utterances and behaviour of people with dementia. We argued that person-centred dementia care education was an attempt to reshape testimonial sensibilities of health and aged care workers. Another way of describing this might be an attempt to widen the "epistemic community". The concept of the epistemic community is helpful in trying to understand the work of patient experience managers and others soliciting digital stories in the context of the Welsh NHS.

Peter Haas (1992) defines epistemic communities as "networks of knowledge based experts" who share values, beliefs about causality, and a common enterprise in their work (Haas, 1992, p. 3). He suggests that they also have "shared notions of validity, that is intersubjective, internally defined criteria for weighing and validating knowledge in their domain of expertise" (Haas, 1992, p. 3). Service improvement projects such as 1000 Lives Plus are, in part, about developing and extending an epistemic community who value patient experiences and stories. This is particularly visible in capacity-building contexts, where, for example, sessions on patient experience are built into corporate inductions for new employees, medical students, or junior doctors, or workshops and guides that offer strategies and ethical guidelines in collecting and using patient stories for service improvement. Haas (1992) recommends considering "the role that networks of knowledge based experts – epistemic communities – play in articulating the cause and effect relationships of complex problems" (p. 2). We would argue that proposing that personal stories are a valuable source of information about the success or otherwise of the NHS, alongside more traditional sources of information such as clinical outcomes, involves epistemic communities reframing complex problems around health.

As Anna Tee points out, listening to digital stories involves quite significant shifts in thinking about what information is important and valid. She comments:

> We're very used to in the NHS a very randomized controlled thing. ... People say "how do you find a representative sample?" And I say "there is no such thing". What stories do is they free you up from that because what you're looking for when you're looking for a story is that person's experience ... You're not looking for them to be representative. I've been a patient, I could only tell a story of my experience, never ever be representative of other people with the same condition. That's the beauty of stories.
>
> (personal communication, patient experience manager, Wales)

Sarah Puntoni comments along similar lines, "No story will ever be representative of all the stories, no experience is representative all experiences, we are all individual; our stories are representative of our own experiences" (personal communication, health improvement lead, Wales).

Even as reports such as Robert et al.'s (2011) *What Matters to Patients?* stress the importance of linking together narratives with other more quantitative types of evidence, Timothy Milewa and Christine Barry (2005) note that "more qualitative or subjective forms of evidence are routinely downplayed by medical professionals and policy-makers" (p. 501). The shift in the epistemic community of health professionals doesn't just involve a change in the way data about clinical safety and effectiveness is viewed, however. It also involves changes in the forms of listening that might be deeply ingrained as part of professional practice. This point is well made by Tee:

> we're expecting people to work in a fundamentally different way to work than they've been in their professions. They've been taught to fix people – that's the premise of their professions. And what I'm coming along and saying is "But you've gotta think about what that feels for somebody at the same time". And that can be a struggle conceptually because it challenges what they've been doing.
>
> (personal communication, patient experience manager, Wales)

Genomics educator and founder of the *Telling Stories* site (NHS National Genetics and Genomics Education Centre, 2014), Maggie Kirk, along with her colleagues, explains how the digital stories on the site challenge nurses and other health care workers to rethink the way they imagine expertise (Kirk et al., 2013). Discussing the use of a mother's story of the fatal consequences of an undiagnosed genetic condition, Professor Kirk describes not just listening, but valuing the information contained in personal narrative and acknowledging the gaps in one's own knowledge, as key professional competencies. She comments:

> There are so many genetic conditions it's quite okay not to know but you need to know that you don't know. You need to know that there may be something going on that you don't know about. ... you need to just listen to what people are telling you and think ... "Is there something I'm missing here?" and also to believe people when they say "something's not right". And people [who] already have a diagnosis tend to be experts in their condition so listen to them as well. You don't have to know it all as the health professional.
>
> (personal communication, genetics educator and academic, Wales)

She adds that a key aim of her teaching is about "being confident in your own professional role, so you are comfortable with not always being the expert and you're comfortable with a family member knowing more than you". The digital narratives on the *Telling Stories* website are intended to convey complex ideas around the science of genomics, but they also work to reframe hierarchies of evidence and generate an epistemic community of careful professional listeners who understand embodied experiential narratives as bearers of critical information.

Patient experience managers we spoke to were involved in expanding an epistemic community that valued and listened to experiential narratives in their roles as facilitators, presenters, and as "listening brokers", finding new opportunities for stories to be heard in induction and in-service training or board meetings. Several people who spoke to us also described developing networks of staff who were not only trained in collecting stories but in thinking through how they might be used. One patient experience manager described her task in training as "to generate a groundswell of people that want to build story in their work" (personal communication, patient experience manager). These networks might be used to train other staff in collecting stories or to brainstorm whether or how stories might be collected and used, as in one manager's "Stories for Improvement" steering group. In developing these networks, patient experience managers were not acting as brokers for particular stories but training others in new ways of valuing and listening to personal narratives. This wasn't an easy task. Resources were a key problem, particularly time. One patient experience manager commented:

> in my ideal world, every service area – if that be a ward, if that be a service, whatever that be – should listen to at least one patient story a year ... you think surely that's not impossible. But that actually doesn't happen.
> (personal communication, patient experience manager, Wales)

"Listenable formats"

All of the practitioners we spoke to were very aware of "classic" or "specific" digital storytelling, and several said they would prefer to collect stories in this way if they had the time and resources. One of the seven Welsh NHS Trusts – the Welsh Ambulance Trust – has a public archive of "specific" digital stories on their website (GIG Cymru & NHS Wales, 2016), generated through participatory workshops. A patient experience manager in a second health trust described "classic" digital stories as the main form used in their work. Others had moved away from "classic" digital storytelling to different modalities of life narrative for diverse, usually quite pragmatic, reasons. While at first glance, these decisions about the story forms seemed driven by resources for story making, we suggest that assumptions and understandings of how the final narratives might be listened to bubble away below the surface. For example, one NHS manager commented:

> We have done some digital stories. The only reason we don't do more digital stories is time and capacity. I'd love to do more. I think they are so

much more powerful when you've got an image of the person or images. I know how to do images. I end up audio editing at home in the evening. It's wrong because it does encroach on my life and that's wrong but that's the reality. When I talk to patients I will. In the majority I do them myself and I don't take them back to patients. I wish I did. There's a part of me that really wishes I could develop like an ongoing relationship with people. But again it's time. I do explain that to the patient at the time.

(personal communication, NHS manager, Wales)

Most trusts relied more on audio or video recordings with the occasional use of written texts. These recordings were often edited for brevity, usually by staff involved in collecting the story.

Others viewed alternative formats for stories as more suitable than "specific" digital storytelling for a range of reasons. Digital stories are used in NHS trusts for a range of purposes, including public information, staff training, and service improvement. One staff member we spoke to commented that using "traditional digital stories … it was really difficult to show a person's [journey]". She noted that some service users, particularly those from marginalised communities, didn't have a collection of personal photographs "and often if they haven't got that they really feel quite awkward because you're asking for something they really haven't got" (personal communication, NHS manager, Wales). She also remarked on the difficulty of finding images that fit with the narratives of screening, diagnosis, and treatment being told. She recalled when "asking them to find pictures to marry up with their stories they'd almost go, 'I don't know what you want', and come with a whole photo book and say, 'What about this? What about this?'" (personal communication, NHS manager, Wales).

While this account might seem to be one about story making, unpinning it are the questions of genres and meanings of domestic photography. There is an interesting tension here between the genre of domestic photography and the kind of narrative of clinical experiences the trust was seeking. Jacqueline Rose's (2010) interviews on the way that British women used family photographs emphasised these women's perception of the role of family photographs in documenting happy times and moments of family togetherness (p. 41). One woman commented to Rose:

I had breast cancer nearly five years ago now, and my husband took a few photos of me with no hair. Obviously didn't go into the family album. I don't know where they are actually. … I mean you don't take photos of sad things. You only take photos of happy things.

(Rose, 2010, p. 13)

Genres of self-representation have expanded in the last decade with the rising popularity of the "selfie", often documenting and sharing the banal and everyday, including the festive, the celebratory, or the "failing" body. Thanks to "Web 2.0", it is now more common to see photographs of ill bodies shared in the public spaces of the media. One common practice here, for example, is sharing photographs of triumphant moments in "the battle against illness", such as the day that cancer survivors finish chemotherapy or the moment they find out that they have "beaten cancer" (Tembeck, 2016). As we discussed in Chapter two, new forms of personal image making, such as those of Angelo and Jennifer Merendino, may include images of painful and uncertain moments during diagnosis and treatment, but such images stand out because of their very rarity. Despite the rise of new genres of image-making, health service users are unlikely to document frightening or worrying engagements with medical and bureaucratic systems like screening and treatment. The challenges of meshing the genres of domestic photography with stories of encounters with biomedical processes could lead to stories where things didn't "work" or make sense, according to staff who spoke to us:

> A story that comes to mind is a lady who went through her experience with us with being diagnosed with breast cancer … throughout that story there were some ups and downs in terms of how her partner coped and whatever. But then with random photographs which really didn't match up with her story that she wanted to use … it was difficult for us to edit it so it did make sense, so it matched up with the narrative.
>
> (personal communication, NHS manager, Wales)

This health trust turned to short videos as an alternative to classic digital storytelling techniques. The mismatch between story and image described here tells us as much about the ways the kind of listening is imagined for these stories as it does about the challenges of finding material to make them.

One of the aims of 1000 Lives Plus was to validate service users' stories as a source of information about patient experience – as we have argued above, broadening out the values of the epistemic community that valued and listened to these types of data. It aimed to attune the ears of staff in the NHS to patient voices, making patient stories listenable – familiar, accepted, or "normal". Ironically, another battle that digital storytelling facilitators and patient experience managers describe was to ensure that the genre of personal narratives did not become so overly familiar or clichéd that they were no longer able to, in story facilitator Lisa Heledd Jones' words, make "the invisible visible" (personal communication).

Autobiographical multimedia narratives have become a very recognisable genre in popular media forms – the video diary in reality TV being one example, or the testimonial interview or video story incorporated into adver-tising. Several of the facilitators and patient experience managers we spoke to saw this very familiarity as a challenge to be navigated in using digital stories within the health system. A digital storytelling facilitator commented on the problems thrown up for those collecting and using digital stories by the affective dimension of charity advertising's use of autobiographical testimony:

There's a lot of people in organisations that say to me that "I don't want to make a '*red nose day*' type story" so. Red Nose Day is a charity in Britain and they raise money for international things … you have these big fund raisers on TV and they're showing Africa and children dying and … also things like using the digital storytelling idea more and more and more, advertising is using it people will say "I don't want to". As soon as it's saying something like "boo hoo", I feel like I'm being forced to feel something – I'm being manipulated.

(personal communication, digital storytelling facilitator, Wales)

Others saw difficulties with adjacent genres of communicating such as the personal testimonial in public relations. One manager working to collect and use stories commented:

What we try as a team to do in terms of we want it raw, we don't want it polished, we don't want it looking corporate … often the challenge for us is trying to get that message across to the organisation. Because organisations by nature … they like everything looking very corporate and glossy and polished! But this it's not about that, is it? This is about people's experience.

(personal communication, NHS manager, Wales)

A patient experience manager discussed her disappointment that a proposal to bring staff stories to a public board, rather than the in-depth story of a particular individual, turned out to be a compilation of sound bites from different staff. She said, "I don't think you'll get the deeper meaning if you just have a soundbite because you just pick up, 'it's fantastic to work here'. I am cynical, I am. You could create a whole positive spin on the organisation" (personal communication, patient experience manager, Wales). The tensions described here reflect some of the ways in which storytelling was mapped in Tee and Gray's (2012) guidance on story collection. Patient stories are seen as having the potential to be used in the media, to combat more negative stories or show that the NHS is taking service improvement seriously. The guidance also points out the value of using stories for "inspiration". What is seen as an ethical imperative to use the valuable narratives of patient experience to their fullest has a more problematic side in the potential for stories being developed and shared as if they were being used for PR purposes.

Like Armstrong and colleagues (2013), the people we spoke to saw standardised or uniform strategies for deploying patient stories as a problem. A patient experience manager in one trust stressed the value of using recorded stories with different levels of "quality" for different purposes – "raw" stories for service improvement and communicating with the public, and more "corporate" versions for publicity. Several of our respondents emphasised the value of using different formats for storytelling to manage the overfamiliarity of personal narratives or their association with spin and corporate communications. These formats included written, audio, and video mediums, as well as innovative strategies such as embedding stories in objects, rather than having them appear in a more familiar manner on screens.

Ethics, editing, and the strategic use of stories

The ways in which the stories are constructed in the Welsh NHS's 1000 Voices Plus project vary significantly from the Center for Digital Storytelling (CDS) model or indeed "specific" digital storytelling more broadly. Key to specific digital storytelling is the idea that the storyteller has control over the editing process. Daniel Meadows, who was key to introducing digital storytelling to Wales via the BBC's (2001–2008) *Capture Wales* program, points out the difference:

> no longer must the public tolerate being "done" by media … no longer must we put up with professional documentarists recording us for hours and then throwing away most of what we tell them, keeping only those bits that tell our stories their own way and, more than likely, at our expense. If we will only learn the skills of Digital Storytelling then we can, quite literally, "take the power back".
>
> (Meadows, 2003, p. 192)

The power of media professionals as mediators is coalesced here in the capacity to edit. The power of editing is equated with a capacity, and perhaps willingness, to harm the storyteller. As we have indicated throughout this book, our understanding of the ways digital stories, broadly understood, work emphasises the inevitability of mediation, which refocuses the meanings of the power to edit in important ways.

Digital storytelling facilitator Lisa Heledd Jones takes on this tricky subject, including traditional "specific" digital storytelling workshops, which she argues involve a collaboration between the facilitator and the storyteller:

> Even if you are getting someone to make their own story in a workshop it's still a collaboration … what you present, what you show them as examples, how you give them feedback on what they've written, all of that is your hand. You can't avoid that.
>
> (personal communication, digital storytelling facilitator, Wales)

She notes that "people don't always want to talk about" this collaborative dimension to "classic" digital storytelling, but argues that this form of collaboration should be celebrated. This perspective on digital storytelling, including "classic" digital storytelling, reframes editing as part of a wider process of collaborative mediation of the story rather than a wresting of control from the storyteller.

Interestingly, our respondents, just like Meadows, stress the importance of the storyteller's ownership in their definition of digital storytelling. However, in explaining the ethics of their approach to editing stories, our respondents stressed the links between the storyteller's ownership of the story, their motive for telling stories, and the editing process. These practitioners certainly didn't see themselves as acting "at the expense" of storytellers, whether others might judge them in this way or not. Rather they explained their choices around editing stories in terms of the ethics of making sure stories were used.

All those we interviewed – digital story facilitators, patient experience managers, and educators using digital stories – agreed that the key rationale for storytellers in the health system is to help others. This was particularly interesting in light of Wang's (2013) analysis of digital storytelling, which suggested that many influential approaches, including that of the CDS, took an "expressivist" view of the value of storytelling – stressing its usefulness for participants and storytellers. Some of our respondents noted the therapeutic value of telling one's story. However, in mapping the motivation of storytellers they stressed the role of altruism (see also Haigh et al., 2014, p. 94).

Heledd Jones commented:

> the idea of you know, of joining a digital storytelling workshop to tell your own story … people feel like it's an egocentric, self involved [… but if] you approach someone and say "We want to tell the stories of chemotherapy … so when people are going to have chemotherapy they know what it's like" they will bite your hand off.
>
> (personal communication, digital storytelling facilitator, Wales)

Given this view of storytellers' motives as primarily about having their stories listened to, our interviewees saw ensuring that storytellers' voices were heard as an ethical duty. Where the registered clinical nursing Clinical Leadership program, from which 1000 Lives Plus drew to generate its story-taking methodology, emphasised that stories should be destroyed after being recorded and analysed, this approach was seen as quite unethical by Sarah Puntoni, for instance:

> Who are we to choose how we are going to use a story? Surely that story is owned by the storyteller. That decision can only be made by the storyteller. But for us to say we're going to take a story, anonymise it, destroy it, is actually quite unethical.
>
> (personal communication, health improvement lead, Wales)

Whereas Meadows (2003) emphasised the violence of editing, Puntoni stresses the danger of not sharing stories, and, like our other respondents, examines the ethics of editing from this starting point. These practitioners believe that it is imperative to use stories, since this is what the owners – the storytellers – want. Our respondents stressed that, "for that story to be used and have a purpose it may need to be edited and shaped." Sarah Puntoni, for instance, felt that it was acceptable to edit a story as long as storytellers were happy "that whoever's going to do that editing understands and is able to portray the key messages" (personal communication, health improvement lead, Wales).

Heledd Jones acknowledged the ethical perils of editing, and in particular, storytellers' concerns that their narrative might just end up "on the cutting room floor". Enabling multiple uses of narratives ensured that she could tell storytellers that "it will get heard" and "there's nothing that they're going to say that isn't going to be useful in some way or another" (personal communication, digital storytelling facilitator, Wales).

All of our interviewees stressed the importance of offering the option to consent to stories being used in a range of contexts before the storytelling began. Heledd Jones described a practice of using a consent form which includes a range of purposes for stories that she is hired to make, film, and facilitate. She suggested that people who were keen to collect stories often hadn't thought through all the possible uses of those stories until they saw the narratives that emerged:

> it's always at the end of the process that people realize the value of what's there and very often they want to use a lot more because then they understand what has been gathered and what people are actually sharing and what's gone into it … people do want to use it but they wouldn't know in advance.
>
> (personal communication, digital storytelling facilitator, Wales)

The practitioners we spoke to were well aware of the implications and possible problems of the editing process. However, the fact that stories should be generated in order to be used was stressed by all of our respondents. Within the service improvement context, an expressivist paradigm of digital storytelling had a limited amount of purchase. A digital storytelling facilitator noted that "if you're working with an organisation that want to train their doctors or whatever, you need to be thinking about what's going to help that doctor hear that thing" (personal communication, digital storytelling facilitator, Wales). Sarah Puntoni commented "stories are a tool … [you can't be too instrumental but] it has to be about what you are trying to achieve" (personal communication, health improvement lead, Wales).

Anna Tee told an interesting story that pointed out the importance of the storyteller driving the narrative and patient experience managers' awareness of the role of editing in reshaping that story. She described a story she "took" in her early years as a patient experience manager. The storyteller:

> talked for the first half about his life, his childhood, about his family, about his farm, about being a county councillor. And I was sitting there thinking "Hmmm. I hope he talks about hospital because if he doesn't what am I going to say??" … But he naturally just went into his hospital story so I didn't have to intervene in any way … [I think] he needed me to

> understand how he was as a person and he needed me to understand who
> he was because when he talked about hospital he talked about really
> being considered as a hip in the bed, the very stereotypical patient things.
>
> (personal communication, patient experience manager, Wales)

She went on to reflect on how that background of his life before the illness, if
included in an edited story, might reshape the responses of listeners, com-
pared to a version which focused on his experiences of hospital. As we discussed in Chapter two, there are powerful arguments for the focusing effect of
concentrating accounts of stories on a person's diagnostic category or illness.
Tee was aware of these effects and had thought through the implications of
the editing she was tasked with doing. While their process was often very
different from "classical" digital storytelling, the difficult balance between an
effective, and purely instrumental, use of stories was one which all our
respondents were closely aware of.

While the format of stories and the way they were collected, edited, and
used in 1000 Lives Plus often diverged quite sharply from "specific" digital
storytelling models, the practitioners we spoke to had very clear definitions of
what was and wasn't a story, which shared many similarities with the CDS
model. Sarah Puntoni stressed the difference between stories on the one hand
and case studies or clinical histories on the other. Anna Tee also described the
challenges of maintaining this distinction in her training sessions. She
suggested that health professionals struggle with stories:

> as a health care professional you've been brought up in a system where
> you're taught to identify a problem and fix it and that's your raison d'etre,
> it's just the way you are and you're hard wired to do that. And when
> you're doing a story you're having to step out of that role because you're
> doing a very, very different role. When you're doing a story you're not
> expected to fix anything. You're not expected to explain or defend, to
> rationalize, to do anything, just to take their story.
>
> (personal communication, patient experience manager, Wales)

Both of these interviewees stressed the importance of experience, the personal,
and feeling:

> if it doesn't have an emotional element, it is not a story. If it doesn't tell
> you what it's like for that person, what the feeling is, what it means to
> them, it is not a story. [... It has to be] personal and it has to have
> something around what matters to them.
>
> (personal communication, patient experience manager, Wales)

> it's about respecting and acknowledging that experience for people as
> being real. Validating that's what happened to somebody.
>
> (personal communication, patient experience manager, Wales)

Heledd Jones, who had acted as a facilitator in a number of Welsh NHS projects, gave a fairly open definition of digital storytelling. She described digital storytelling as "personal narratives presented in some digital form where that person feels ownership over their story" (personal communication, digital storytelling facilitator, Wales). Heledd Jones' working method didn't always involve storytellers editing stories. However, she saw a critical element of ownership as the content and general direction of the story being led by the storyteller. Even when she was asked to pull together a compilation of stories around a theme, she saw this as a digital storytelling, "because it's still whatever their experience is of that thing. Even if [there is a defined] theme of what we're looking at, they could still choose where we go with that." She contrasted this to what she called "films", which may still incorporate personal narratives:

> If it's like a film of six different voices in it all of people who've experienced mental health but the end result of it needs to be that the big thing that has helped them is coming to this support group and that is what the film is for is to encourage people to come to the support group then I wouldn't call that a digital story, because even if they had shared all kinds of things with me, I'm going to be choosing the bits that are to do with the story. ... because the ownership isn't theirs. They could say "I don't want that bit in" but they can't really say "can you keep that thing in about my" ... well, you could, I'd probably try and fit anything they particularly wanted in but it's ... not led by them.
>
> (personal communication, digital storytelling facilitator, Wales)

Theorising listening: the emotional and the everyday

Emotion and unlearning

The affective power of personal stories illustrated by images is often seen as key to the impact of digital stories. Work on service user involvement in decision-making in the NHS has suggested, for example, that patient stories can encourage emotional engagement by health professionals; part of what Mary Dixon-Woods, Sarah McNicol, and Graham Martin (2012) see as a key benefit of stories in the context of quality improvement. Natalie Armstrong and her colleagues (2013) have summarised this notion of using the patient voice as a "technology of persuasion". Patient Voices, a pre-eminent exemplar of the use of digital stories in service improvement in the UK, also emphasises the role of "affecting stories" in mobilising staff to change practice (Stabler, 2014, p. 172).

As we saw in Chapter three, practitioners using digital stories in professional education see the emotional power of stories as potentially valuable, but also potentially dangerous. In the context of dementia education, heartbreaking stories were seen as potentially off-putting to new recruits in health and medicine in the distinctly unsexy field of gerontology. While practitioners valued moving stories as a pedagogical resource, they also saw it as a potential threat to engagement and learning.

Our interviews suggested a similar ambivalence about emotional digital storytelling in the context of service improvement. One respondent articulated the possible dangers of digital stories: "You have to be careful. Your duty of care in presenting a story is not just to the patient and storyteller, also to the people that are going to listen" (patient experience manager, Wales). Another argued that heightened emotion in stories could shut down listening, rather than allowing staff to connect to the underlying narrative. She notes:

> if you start crying as well … you've lost people when you start crying because you can't hear anything, and people think "I've got to create a bubble to preserve my sanity now, I can't manage this." You know, none of us can deal with stuff when we're emotionally distraught, in our lives.
> (patient experience manager, Wales)

Rushmer and Davies (2004) in their consideration of the role of "unlearning" – changing established practices and understandings by no longer doing things – offered some useful perspectives on the affective power of digital storytelling in health. They argued that, "Unlearners may experience powerful negative emotions, such as blame, shame, guilt, fear, and rage. These emotions may cause harm if not worked through. Unlearners may also experience something akin to mourning, and start a grieving cycle" (Rushmer & Davies, 2004, pp. ii14–ii15; see also Stabler, 2014).

Anna Tee told us a story that highlighted the dangers associated with the emotional power of digital storytelling. She described a nurse preceptor training session, in which newly qualified nurses were mentored and supported in their roles. After screening a particular story, two of the new nurses burst into tears, and had to be calmed down by the trainer and teacher. According to Tee, the conflict between their "good intentions" as nurses, and the reality of what they felt able to do under existing constraints, was brought into painful focus by the experience of watching a story about poor patient experiences. This patient experience manager described the necessity of managing these reactions and suggested the need to map out coping strategies. She felt that people using patient stories should be clear to their audiences that there is a "possibility that this will increase your frustration. You'll hear that patients talking about what you want to do" (personal communication, patient experience manager, Wales). Stanton, discussing the use of patient stories in service improvement, observed that "ambivalence and sometimes aggressive / defensive responses" can be evoked from professionals listening to patient stories. He suggested that such responses can be located in "the exercise of unquestioned authority and control" that medical staff are accustomed to in their work (Stanton, 2014, p. 58). The observations of the people we spoke to in patient experience management and other "listening broker" positions suggested that the inversion of the hierarchy between expert and patient was far from the only reason for emotional or defensive responses from staff to hearing patient voices.

This highlights the potential for digital stories that aim to improve service delivery and outcomes to precipitate value conflict for staff. If, as Michael Lipsky (1980) has argued, professional work under imperfect circumstances often leads to staff developing a "cognitive shield" so as not to be constantly and painfully aware of the contradictions between the values they profess and the professional practice they might adopt, Anna Tee's story suggests a way that digital stories might serve to pull down that cognitive shield for some staff. This may be a fine opportunity for learning.

Tony Sumner of Pilgrim Projects describes this process well:

> So [for] a lot of viewers of the stories, they – there is a resistant response, because they are emotionally affected by the stories, in some way or other. They're not playing vanilla instructional videos. This is what happens, this should happen. So there will always be some level of resistant response, I think. ... But I think some people that respond – they manage to surf the wave and they ride on top of that emotional thing. It carries them forward. Some people stand firm against it.
> (personal communication, digital storytelling facilitator, England)

If, as we discussed in Chapter three, drawing on the work of Megan Boler (1999), testimonial listening involves acknowledgement of your own implication in the difficulties described in the story you are listening to, the digital story Anna Tee used in this training session seemed to prompt this kind of listening, which Boler sees as very valuable. However, as the response of the listeners makes clear, this was not a painless process.

Some strategies for addressing the emotional labour of listening to stories were suggested by the practitioners we spoke to. One was to draw on stories that had less explicit messages, requiring reflection by the listening health practitioner. Paul Stanton (2014) argues that the "poetic qualities" of Patient Voices digital stories – multisensory, affecting, but also their being open to interpretation – enable them to provoke reflection. He notes that Patient Voices stories don't so much provide answers about providing expert care or governance, but "help individual professionals and clinical teams to formulate ever more thoughtful and focused questions" (Stanton, 2014, p. 64)

The storytelling facilitators and participation brokers we have spoken to, working with stories in both education and service improvement contexts, have suggested the value of stories that leave space for the listener to reflect and make active connections to their own experience, rather than having the meaning of the story fully nailed down, or blame explicitly evoked. In Chapter three, we heard from dementia trainers that "pausable" stories were particularly valuable – ones where workers could think through what they might have done themselves or how they would have reacted in the situation being described. Stories might be constructed to allow testimonial listening – to allow the listener to consider how they themselves might be implicated in the predicament the story describes. Effective stories, according to Heledd Jones, for instance, are about "making the dramas smaller, making it more positive" (personal communication, digital storytelling facilitator, Wales).

All of our respondents stressed the importance of little things in constructing the patient experience – from introducing oneself, through to taking the time to hold a patient's hand. One patient experience manager we talked to described this as "about making small changes, because we're not talking about massive changes, we're talking about small changes which make a big difference to somebody using the service" (patient experience manager, Wales). "Small stories", in the words of one digital storytelling facilitator, are often seen as the most helpful for making these small changes. This emphasis on "sweating the small stuff" also emerged from Locock et al.'s (2014) research using narratives from the *HealthTalkOnline* (DIPEx, 2016) archive for service improvement.

Pip Hardy told us an interesting story about defensiveness in the reception of digital stories. She described one of the earliest stories she and Tony Sumner pulled together for the National Audit Office, entitled "Thank you very much" (Lett, n.d.). This "classic" digital story was made by Vanessa Lett, about the birth and care of her premature baby girl, Evie. The story tells a tale of her daughter's unexpectedly early birth, the hospital's difficulty in finding a humidicrib for Evie, and subsequent medical errors, when Evie was given a massive overdose of anaesthetic during heart surgery. However, as Hardy described, "at the end of the story, it's a beautiful … story. She says basically, Evie's now nine months old, she's lovely, we love her to pieces, and thank you very much for our baby" (personal communication, digital storytelling facilitator, England).

Part of Vanessa's voice-over illustrates Hardy's point about upbeat story tone. She described Evie's progress at nine months old:

> She's so content and happy. This I think is due to the care she received. We cannot express the care and love that Evie received from each one of the nurses that she came into contact with. When we came home … the level of care we received was fantastic as well. We had outreach nurses ringing us, visiting us, as often as we wanted. We had dieticians looking after Evie's nutritional needs, who would ring, just to see if everything was okay, and generally it was … they gave us all the information we needed for benefits, for help, because she did need special care, they made sure we were never left with questions unanswered. Continuity of care was outstanding.
>
> (Lett, n.d.)

Pip Hardy described a very different interpretation of this story by its organisational audience:

What the people in the public accounts committee said was, this was a terrible story. This is an awful, bad news [story] criticising the hospital, criticising the doctors, and – but it wasn't. It was just telling her story, and then it was a story of gratitude.

(personal communication, digital storytelling facilitator, England)

Hardy's account of the reception of this story is instructive, suggesting that even a generally positive story like this can be interpreted as being negative by the commissioning organisation. Hardy comments that this is not an uncommon experience for *Patient Stories*:

People quite often will email us and say, all the stories on your website are so miserable. Haven't you got any good news stories? We think – well, actually, most of them are good news stories. ... there is something about people hearing what they want to hear.

(personal communication, digital storytelling facilitator, England)

Placing stories: locating stories within organisations

Within "classic" digital storytelling practice, a great deal is vested in the universality of digital stories and their ability to speak across differences. Stories are often said to be "timeless" (Hardy & Sumner, 2014; O'Neill, 2014; Taylor & Hardy, 2014) and able to be reused in many different contexts. Hardy and Sumner, for example, memorably refer to Patient Voices digital stories as "reusable atomic learning objects" (personal communication, digital storytelling facilitators, England). In our conversations, there have been mixed responses to such arguments. Patient experience manager Anna Tee, for instance, stresses that the key themes of stories are not necessarily connected to specific contexts of care. She remarked, with some amazement:

I've listened to stories across all the different types of care that we provide and they're so similar, they're so, so similar. They might talk about different specific experiences and different clinical conditions but the themes of what people say are consistent.

(personal communication, patient experience manager, England)

Perhaps as a consequence, she argues that stories from other locations can sometimes work better to defuse defensiveness than stories from "here":

I'll say to people, I'm consciously bringing you a story from another area and I will explain that the reason that I'm doing that is if the first story I bring you is from your area, I can guarantee you will get massively defensive and you will shut down and you won't hear what is trying to be said. And I tell them that up front. So I say, I'll bring you a story from another area, so you'll feel completely safe to criticize, condemn, praise, whatever it is, but you'll feel more able to talk about it. So they understand what they're going to hear in the story. And it doesn't happen like that all the time, but that's my ideal situation. And then I find that they want to hear a story from their own area then because they're more receptive because they get it then.

(personal communication, patient experience manager, England)

Locock and colleagues (2014), in their rich study of the ways in which health care narratives can be used to prompt patient–professional co-production of change in the health care system, agreed that locally produced narratives were not necessarily essential to prompt change. Their research, like ours, concludes that the potentially confronting accounts of poor practice can be thought through less defensively and more fruitfully by staff when the stories emerge from another location.

If the themes of stories are often shared, their effectivity is often seen as fundamentally connected to particular locations and the sensory experience of place. One patient experience manager observed:

And last year I said "Isn't it brilliant that hospitals don't smell any more!" and they promptly reminded me that they did still smell but I had lost the ability to smell them. And that was really powerful for me. I thought if I can't smell what's really there, then what else do I not see, do I not feel … one of the best things you can do day to day to improve your life is every now and again just stop … maybe not in the middle of doing something … ·stand at the edge of where you work, and just observe – look and hear and smell and feel, just for five minutes just actively build that into your practice so you constantly have a reminder of what is it like to be a patient here.

(personal communication, patient experience manager, Wales)

The philosophy of 1000 Lives Plus has been to embed capability for story collection and use across the different health care trusts in Wales, rather than having a central archive or collection point for stories. Sarah Puntoni says that "stories should be collected and listened to by everyone" (personal communication, health improvement lead, Wales). She emphasises the importance of a range of different staff collecting stories: not just nurses, who often have training in storytelling collection through the RCN Clinical Leadership program, but everyone from doctors to porters. However, she acknowledged that "in reality" collecting and particularly editing stories "mostly rests with the patient experience manager" (personal communication, health improvement lead, Wales).

This disseminated approach to collecting patient stories is connected to an understanding of service improvement as happening locally:

The whole point of collecting stories is for improvement. If I collect a story centrally I have very little room to make an improvement based on that story at a local level. What I can do is use it as a communication tool, what I can't do is force a change at a local level.

(patient experience manager, Wales)

Just like the dementia trainers we discussed in Chapter three, some patient experience managers deliberately chose to make the connection between a story and the professional practice of people in the session clear and obvious when deciding which stories to use in training. In short periods of in-service or induction training, we heard that staff often need to have it made very clear to them "how does what I'm hearing ... relate to my job?" (personal communication, patient experience manager, Wales).

The idea of patient experience of care – and professional dispositions and practices – emerging from an environment, and consequently digital story-telling having its effects in a particular environment is a powerful one. Our interviewees downplayed the significance of individual intention in negative patient experiences. One patient experience manager commented:

Nobody comes into work in the morning and they're thinking in their car in the morning, "do you know today I know what I'm going to do I'm going to leave all the food out of their reach, I'm going to make sure they dehydrate" but there's something that when they work in the system that creates that environment.

(personal communication, patient experience manager, Wales)

This listening "broker" explicitly points out that practices that can lead to bad patient experience are "not actually conscious thought" (personal communication). She remarked, "Some of it is attitude but then I think you can also trace that attitude back to the system." The unit of analysis for failures of care is not necessarily the individual person, their ethics, or their insights. Rather, it's the organisation.

Jane Bennett's (2010) discussion of responsibility in the context of failures of complex systems or assemblages that incorporate human action, objects, and practices is useful here. Rather than thinking about digital stories as untethered and individual, our fieldwork has suggested that stories are viewed as being most powerful in particular locations – framed in particular ways, contextualised, and located.

Bennett (2010) argued that individual human agency is not always the best way of thinking through why things happen, or indeed, allocating blame when things go wrong. She cited Noortje Marres' comment, "it is often hard to grasp just what the sources of agency are that make a particular event happen" and that this "ungraspability may be an [essential] aspect of agency" (Bennett, 2010, p. 36). She suggests that:

Outrage will not and should not disappear, but a politics devoted too exclusively to moral condemnation and not enough to a cultivated

discernment of the web of agentic capacities can do little good. A mor-
alized politics of good and evil, of singular agents who must be made to
pay for their sins ... becomes unethical.

(Bennett, 2010, p. 38)

Storytelling facilitator, Lisa Heledd Jones, gives a great example of the way in
which patient experience is disseminated and located, tied to the idea of
stories as being most effectively embedded in particular places. She described
an audio recording made by a breast cancer survivor as she walked around
the hospital where she was treated. Heledd Jones described one of the nine
vignettes that made up the storywalk:

> there's a story about a beep. And it's a beep that happens overnight and a
> machine is broken and no one on the shift can fix it and they have to wait
> for someone. And the feelings and the anxiety this builds in her ... [but]
> never a complaint would have been made. ... Then having shown it to the
> person who looks after the machines his response was "Oh we can get
> people to learn how to fix that, that isn't a problem. We didn't know that
> was a problem. We didn't know that these machines were going off at
> night." And again it's a tiny thing. Huge overall impact.
> (personal communication, digital storytelling facilitator, Wales)

The story, in Heledd Jones' account, is part of an individual digital story. But
it's also about a beep, and the machine that goes beep, and about the staff at
night who don't know how to fix it, and the man who fixes it, but doesn't
know it goes off in the night. The effect of the story is not necessarily about
individuals taking responsibility or being more aware of patients' needs. It is
about the way systems play out in particular places and particular times.
Heledd Jones' strategy for using the story, to get staff at the hospital to hear
the story in the place where the patient experienced that errant beep, also
emphasises places and relationships as part of the potential effectiveness of
ways of learning and relearning. We are a long way here from a disembodied
one-to-one model of dissemination of stories. According to the people we
spoke to, effectively changing practice is about locating stories in particular
places – social contexts as well as physical locations. Rushmer and Davies
(2004) frame such processes in terms of organisational memory. They suggest
that "organisations are inanimate entities, but they do have ways of capturing,
recording, and reproducing what they know" (Rushmer & Davies, 2004, p.
ii12). Changing practices then means organisations, not just the individuals
within them, doing the difficult work of unlearning.

Take-aways for practitioners

- When considering how digital stories might be used, think about the ethical
  implications of not using stories, as well as the risks of using them.

- When brokering listening for service improvement contexts, bear in mind the possible emotional challenges of unlearning old practices.
- Given the varied political origins of the push towards public and patient involvement in health, don't assume that resistance to hearing patient voices reflects an expectation of unquestioned authority.
- Stories that open up opportunities for professionals to pose questions and consider alternative actions or interventions, rather than having a very clear "message", may be valuable in promoting change.
- In selecting stories to use, consider whether listeners may interpret them as examples of public relations or corporate communications.
- Consider using a variety of forms of personal narrative to provoke fresh listening.

Conclusion

The political meanings of the uses organisations made of storytelling are complicated. Our interviewees might be described using Harrison and Mort's (1998) term "participation entrepreneurs" or Li and colleagues' (2015) expression "public involvement brokers". They were neither senior members of the NHS bureaucracy nor "grassroots" staff, but people, in one respondent's words, "in the middle of the sandwich". Such mediators are seen by Li and colleagues (2015) as key to the ways in which participant interventions in health are used. Our respondents could be understood both as actively seeking to shift existing medical hierarchies by drawing on and amplifying the voices of health service users, and as the "insiders" to the NHS negotiating demands for participation and new political priorities. They reported navigating and sometimes speaking back to biomedically focused traditions in the health services, in which non-clinical staff may be viewed as less authoritative than health professionals. At the same time, they had a strong investment in the health service of which they are a part. As Li and colleagues (2015) map out, for such public involvement brokers "conflicts may arise as decision-makers navigate their accountabilities to their organization and to their new allegiances to public involvement participants" (p. 19).

The frank and fascinating interviews our participants provided, speaking to us as researchers, could be viewed in many ways as embodying and enacting the demand for a culture of openness in the NHS, of which patient storytelling is a part. A case study around the Welsh Ambulance Health Trust's (WAST) use of "specific" digital stories notes that by its use of stories in public spaces like the Trust's website "where there have been negative experiences, we can demonstrate that WAST has an open culture and is a Trust that puts the patient's experience at the heart of service development and improvement" (Puntoni et al. 2012, p. 6). The openness of the 1000 Lives Plus project, the fact that so many of its guidance and policy documents are up on the web for anyone to see, was repeatedly emphasised in interviews. This is not to say that we can think of our interview materials as simply public relations. Several of our interviewees commented on the tensions between the various uses of stories – for education or service improvement on the one hand and for public relations or media purposes on the other. They acknowledged that sometimes organisations seek to, in Harrison and Mort's (1998) words, "[play the] user card" (p. 66), while explaining that their own activities in the organisation are not about this. The people we spoke to who worked within the NHS described themselves as being in a complex relationship with the bureaucracy around them, at times feeling required to defend it against critics, while at the same time being very aware of its limitations and flaws. These issues, we feel, simply give us a layer of richness to add in thinking about the way digital storytelling is used in organisations.

Our focus in this chapter has been on mapping the way that digital stories might be used as a tool for improving primary and acute health care services. In Chapter five we will extend and further think through the conclusion to this chapter – that is, that listening to digital storytelling for service improvement is best conceptualised as embodied and located, in organisations and in particular spaces.

References

Armstrong, N., Herbert, G., Aveling, E., Dixon-Woods, M., & Martin, G. (2013). Optimizing patient involvement in quality improvement. *Health Expectations, 16*(3), e36–47.

BBC (2001–2008). *Capture Wales*. Retrieved from http://www.bbc.co.uk/wales/audiovi deo/sites/galleries/pages/capturewales.shtml

Bennett, J. (2010). *Vibrant Matter: A Political Ecology of Things*. Durham, NC: Duke University Press.

Boler, M. (1999). *Feeling Power: Emotions and Education*. Hove: Psychology Press.

Davies, H., Powell, A., & Rushmer, R. (2007). Why don't clinicians engage with quality improvement? *Journal of Health Service Research and Policy, 12*(3), 129–130.

DIPEx (2016). *Health Talk Online* [Website]. Retrieved from http://www.healthtalk.org/

Dixon-Woods, M., McNicol, S., & Martin, G. (2012). Ten challenges in improving quality in healthcare: Lessons from the Health Foundation's evaluations and relevant literature. *BMJ Quality and Safety, 21*(10), 876–884.

Dyer, S., McDowell, L., & Banitzky, A. (2008). Emotional labour/body work: The caring labours of migrants in the UK's National Health Service. *Geoforum, 39*(6), 2030–2038.

Francis, R. (2013). *The Mid Staffordshire NHS Foundation Trust. Report of the Mid Staffordshire NHS Foundation Trust Public Inquiry. Executive Summary*. Retrieved from http://webarchive.nationalarchives.gov.uk/20150407084003/http://www.midsta ffspublicinquiry.com/report

Fricker, M. (2003). Epistemic injustice and a role for virtue in the politics of knowing. *Metaphilosophy, 34*(1–2), 154–173.

GIG Cymru & NHS Wales (2016). *Welsh Ambulance Services Trust* [Website]. Retrieved from http://www.was-tr.wales.nhs.uk/

Haas, P. M. (1992). Epistemic communities and international policy coordination. *International Organization, 46*(1), 1–35.

Haigh, C., Cahoon, P., & Sumner, T. (2014). Working with dignity and respect: Improving mental health services. In P. Hardy & T. Sumner (Eds.), *Cultivating Compassion: How Digital Storytelling is Transforming Healthcare* (pp. 87–96). Chichester: Kingsham Press.

Hardy, P., & Sumner, T. (Eds.) (2014). *Cultivating Compassion: How Digital Storytelling is Transforming Healthcare.* Chichester: Kingsham Press.

Harrison, S., & Mort, M. (1998). Which champions? Which people? Public and user involvement in health care as a technology of legitimation. *Social Policy and Administration, 32*(1), 60–70.

Heywood, T., Puntoni, S., & Spencer, M. (2012). *Face to Face Storytelling at a Board Meeting. Patient and Person Driven Care, Case Study – No. 3.* Retrieved from http://www.1000livesplus.wales.nhs.uk/sitesplus/documents/1011/Stories%20Case%20Study%20No%20%203%20%2D%20C%26V%20face%20to%20face%20storytelling%20at%20Board%20meetings%20%28Final%29.pdf

Kirk, M., Tonkin, E., Skirton, H., McDonald, K., Cope, B., & Morgan, R. (2013). Storytellers as partners in developing a genetics education resource for health rofessionals. *Nurse Education Today, 33*(5), 518–524.

Kvarnstrom, S. (2011). *Collaboration in Health and Social Care. Service User Participation and Teamwork in Interprofessional Clinical Microsystems* (Doctoral dissertation). Jonkoping, Sweden:Jonkoping University. Retrieved from https://www.diva-portal.org/smash/get/diva2:417626/FULLTEXT01.pdf

Lett, V. (n.d.). Thank you very much. *Patient Voices.* http://www.patientvoices.org.uk/flv/0142pv384.htm

Li, K., Abelson, J., Giacomini, M., & Contandriopoulos, D. (2015). Conceptualizing the use of public involvement in health policy decision-making. *Social Science & Medicine, 138,* 14–21.

Lipsky, M. (1980). *Street-level Bureaucracy: Dilemmas of the Individual in Public Services.* New York: Sage.

Locock, L., Robert, G., Boaz, A., Vougioukalou, S., Shuldham, C., Fielden, J., Ziebland, S., Gager, M., Tollyfield, R., & Pearcey, J. (2014). Using a national archive of patient experience narratives to promote local patient-centered quality improvement: An ethnographic process evaluation of 'accelerated' experience-based co-design. *Journal of Health Services Research & Policy, 19*(4), 200–207.

Martin, G. (2008). 'Ordinary people only': Knowledge, representativeness, and the publics of public participation in healthcare. *Sociology of Health & Illness, 30*(1), 35–54.

Martin, G., McKee, L., & Dixon-Woods, M. (2015). Beyond metrics? Utilizing 'soft intelligence' for healthcare quality and safety. *Social Science & Medicine, 142,* 19–26.

Meadows, D. (2003). Digital storytelling: Research-based practice in new media. *Visual Communication, 2*(2), 189–193.

Milewa, T., & Barry, C. (2005). Health policy and the politics of evidence. *Social Policy and Administration, 39*(5), 498–512.

National Advisory Group on the Safety of Patients in England (2013). *A Promise to Learn – a Commitment to Act. Improving the Safety of Patients in England.* Retrieved from https://www.gov.uk/government/publications/berwick-review-into-patient-safety

NHS National Genetics and Genomics Education Centre (2014). *Telling Stories. Understanding Real Life Genetics* [Website]. Retrieved from http://www.tellingstories.nhs.uk/

NHS Wales (n.d.). *1000 Lives Plus* [Website]. Retrieved from http://www.1000livesplus. wales.nhs.uk/home

O'Neill, F. (2014). Arthur and Co: Digital stories of arthritis. In P. Hardy & T. Sumner (Eds.), *Cultivating Compassion: How Digital Storytelling is Transforming Healthcare* (pp. 67–76). Chichester: Kingsham Press.

Pilgrim Projects (2016). *Patient Voices* [Website]. Retrieved from http://www.patient voices.org.uk/

Puntoni, S., Hawker, L., Sullivan, H., & Clement, A. (2012). Collecting and sharing stories via the Welsh Ambulance Services Trust website. *Patient and Person Driven Care Case Study No. 1, 1000 Lives Plus* (pp. 1–11). NHS Wales. Retrieved from http://www.1000livesplus.wales.nhs.uk/sitesplus/documents/1011/Stories%20Case% 20Study%20No%20%201%20%2D%20WAST%20%28Final%29.pdf

Renedo, A., Marston, C. A., Spyridonidis, D., & Barlow, J. (2015). Patient and public involvement in healthcare quality improvement: How organizations can help patients and professionals to collaborate. *Public Management Review, 17*(1), 17–34.

Robert, G., Cornwell, J., Brearley, S., Foot, C., Goodrich, J., Joule, N., Levenson, R., Maben, J., Murrells, T., Tsianakas, V., & Waite, D. (2011). *What Matters to Patients? Developing the Evidence Base for Measuring and Improving Patient Experience. Project Report for the Department of Health and NHS Institute for Innovation & Improvement.* Retrieved from http://www.institute.nhs.uk/patient_exp erience/guide/the_patient_experience_research.html

Rose, G. (2010). *Doing Family Photography: The Domestic, the Public and the Politics of Sentiment.* Farnham: Ashgate.

Rushmer, R., & Davies, H. T. O. (2004). Unlearning in health care. *Quality & Safety in Health Care, 13*(Suppl. II), ii10–ii15.

Spencer, M., Puntoni, S., & Matthias, J. (2015). *Listening and Learning to Improve the Experience of Care. Understanding What it Feels Like to Use Services in NHS Wales. Improving Health Care White Paper Series – No. 14. GIG Cymru & NHS Wales.* Retrieved from http://www.1000livesplus.wales.nhs.uk/listening-and-learning

Stabler, A. (2014). Healthy teams: The challenge of implementing digital storytelling in healthcare organisations. In P. Hardy & T. Sumner (Eds.), *Cultivating Compassion: How Digital Storytelling is Transforming Healthcare* (pp. 165–174). Chichester: Kingsham Press.

Stanton, P. (2014). Towards compassionate governance: The impact of Patient Voices on NHS leadership. In P. Hardy & T. Sumner (Eds.), *Cultivating Compassion: How Digital Storytelling is Transforming Healthcare* (pp. 55–66). Chichester: Kingsham Press.

Stewart, E. (2011). *Governance, Participation and Avoidance: Everyday Public Invol-vement in the Scottish National Health Service.* PhD thesis. Edinburgh: University of Edinburgh.

Taylor, K., & Hardy, P. (2014). Measuring what counts: Digital stories as qualitative data. In P. Hardy & T. Sumner (Eds.), *Cultivating Compassion: How Digital Storytelling is Transforming Healthcare* (pp. 175–184). Chichester: Kingsham Press.

Tee, A., & Gray, J. (2012). *Learning to Use Patient Stories. Tools for Improvement 6. GIG Cymru & NHS Wales.* Retrieved from http://www.1000livesplus.wales.nhs.uk/ stories

Tembeck, T. (2016). Selfies of ill health: Online autopathographic photography and the dramaturgy of the everyday. *Social Media and Society, 2*(1), 1–11.

Topol, E. (2015). *The Patient Will See You Now. The Future of Medicine is in Your Hands*. New York: Basic Books.

Tovey, P., Atkin, K., & Milewa, T. (2001). The individual and primary care: Service user, reflexive choice maker and collective actor. *Critical Public Health, 11*(2), 153–166.

Wang, X. (2013). *A Genre Theory Perspective on Digital Storytelling*. PhD thesis. Nashville, TN: Vanderbilt University.

5 Listening in community and place-based health promotion

In this chapter we step out of acute individual-oriented health care and education settings to explore digital storytelling and listening in community and place-based health promotion settings. These settings are widely recognised as shaping meso-level social and environmental determinants of health, which in turn shape individual factors and outcomes. Storytelling researchers and practitioners from the fields of media and cultural studies, and narrative inquiry, have long recognised the dialogic and relational nature of storytelling and listening, that is, the complex, dynamic, and often fluid relationships between storytellers and listeners and the acts of listening to and telling a story. In order to extend current thinking on listening, we suggest that listening also occurs in a complex and fluid dialogue with our embodied and emplaced experiences and ways of knowing. We explore this concept of embodied and emplaced listening through a case study of storytelling work with children and young people in Australia.

Dialogic storytelling and listening in context

Before we introduce the concept of embodied and emplaced listening in this chapter we will first recap current understandings about the way listening is embedded in social, cultural, and community settings. This includes understanding the embeddedness of storytelling and listening within interpersonal relationships between storytellers and listeners as well as broader social, cultural, political, and geographical systems. For over two decades, narrative researchers (see for example, Clandinin & Connelly, 2000; Connelly & Clandinin, 1990; Kim, 2016) have underlined the dialogic and deeply interpersonal nature of storytelling and listening, emphasising the two-way construction of stories between the storyteller and listener(s). The "inter-subjective" view of narrative and stories in narrative inquiry recognises both the interpretive nature of storytelling and listening and the role that others play in helping us to extend our stories through social interactions and relationships, for example, through questioning, reciprocal story sharing, and trust building. Some studies of storytelling and listening, in psychology for example – which tend perhaps more towards "conversational analysis" – have emphasised that listener responses to narrative – for instance, whether the listener is attentive or distracted – intimately affect the ways stories are told and ways in which meaning is communicated (Bavelas, Coates, & Johnson, 2000). Bavelas et al. (2000) are among many interdisciplinary narrative researchers who assert that listeners should be seen as "co-narrators" of the resulting story's meanings and implications for action and reaction. While this recognition of the listener as co-narrator has occurred in narrative inquiry, the role of the listener has been less overtly recognised in the digital storytelling literature and related research. Despite this, productive overlaps exist between narrative inquiry and digital storytelling, particularly in relation to how we recognise the role of the listener and the unavoidable movement of meanings that occurs through mediation and listening.

Narrative researchers' recognition of the role of the listener and the dialogic co-creation of stories between tellers and listeners has been significantly influenced by the theoretical traditions that inform their approach. Narrative researchers assume that humans make sense of their lives through the repeated telling and listening of stories at both the individual and collective levels. According to this view, an individual's stories are shaped by the collective's – what are often called meta-narratives – and vice versa. Hence, drawing on a range of theoretical traditions, including in particular social constructivism and poststructuralism, Connelly and Clandinin (1990) have emphasised the many steps of storying and restorying that can occur between the story "teller" and the "listener". This fluid and dialogic view of storytelling and listening acknowledges in particular the mediation that inevitably occurs in every act of storytelling and listening as we outlined in Chapter one. Narrative research methodologies then often include numerous waves of participant storytelling, researcher listening, researcher interpretation of stories, and feedback loops in an attempt to ensure that researchers have adequately "heard" the stories that participants want to tell. Through this process of dialogic storying, listening, and interpreting, new stories and new or expanded *versions* of previously told stories can also emerge. The narrative research process of storying, interpreting, checking, restorying, and listening hence pays respect to both the *dialogic* and inherently *dynamic* nature of storytelling and listening in social relationships.

Storytelling and listening in social, political, and cultural contexts

Alongside the theoretical traditions that have informed narrative inquiry, critical and emancipatory theoretical approaches have been used extensively in both digital storytelling and social models of health and well-being. As outlined in Chapter one, experiences of oppression and marginalisation are fundamental determinants of health and well-being not just for those who are directly disadvantaged but for all people in unequal societies (Wilkinson & Pickett, 2009). An extensive body of evidence internationally shows that more unequal societies exhibit higher rates of illiteracy, unwanted teenage pregnancy, incarceration, unemployment, and violent crime (see for example, Krug, Mercy, Dahlberg & Zwi, 2002; Reading & Wien, 2009; Wilkinson & Marmot, 2003): all of which are determinants of health in and of themselves. Consequently, we maintain that it is in health and social policy makers' and practitioners' – as well as digital story proponents', participants', and researchers' – interests to understand the political realities and limits, as well as the potential, of digital storytelling and listening within the context of current dominant systems of privilege and oppression. Any attempt to understand the ultimate social justice impact of digital storytelling which doesn't take into account these existing systems of privilege and oppression in contemporary societies will be at best naïve and at worst reproduce practices and experiences of oppression and marginalisation.

As we have noted throughout the book, experienced digital storytelling practitioners are acutely aware of the way storytelling unfolds in political, cultural, and social contexts. In Chapter four, for example, we discussed the tensions that emerged for patient experience managers in the British National Health Service as they solicited and used stories as a way of shaping service provision in primary health care. Likewise, narrative researchers have deeply questioned the power relationships involved in the co-construction of narrative in narrative research, and the ethics of such interactions. This is particularly the case where researchers feel that there is a power imbalance between themselves and participant narrators due to, for example, unfamiliarity between the researchers and participants, the researcher's social privilege, or unequal control of research processes, resources, and outcomes. Simply acknowledging the co-construction of stories does not somehow remove storytelling, either in research or public health contexts, from this terrain of power. However, the work done in interrogating the ethics of the complex mediations of life stories by narrative researchers allows us to think about these power relations in terms that move beyond simplistic binaries of control and lack of control; autonomy and its opposite; ownership of a story and loss of ownership. A deep understanding of this complexity has been evident in the conversations we have had with digital storytelling practitioners, but this nuance is not always evident in the published literature in the field, with its emphasis on the value of digital storytelling as a tool of empowerment.

Once again, we observe that inquirers and theorists outside of specific digital storytelling can offer much to our shared understanding of the social, political, and cultural shaping of digital storytelling and listening. Narrative theorists such as Kristin Langellier (1989) for example have emphasised that "personal narratives are locally occasioned in conversations as participants 'do' their talk and their relationships in everyday life" (p. 256) and that "storytelling is embedded within larger social processes" (p. 261). This recognition of social "context" has a number of dimensions that are conceptually relevant to the current chapter. First, personal narratives are constructed in dialogue with broader shared social narratives relating to identity, place, and experience. In this way, personal narratives can be seen as "collaborative social enactments of individual, relational, and public identities" (Beck, 2005, p. 61). An individual's narrative is not only created in dialogue with immediate and present "listeners", but also in dialogue with broader social "meta-narratives" and stereotypes about, for example, "people like me/us" who inhabit "places like this". In her later work Langellier (2011) referred to the act of "performing" narrative to emphasise the role of the individual storyteller in reproducing meta-narratives that are produced and circulated over time through many and varied processes of cultural and social transmission. Langellier (1989) asserts that "all personal narratives are ideological because they evolve from a structure of power relations and simultaneously produce, maintain and reproduce that power structure" (p. 267).

Langellier's account of personal narrative as emerging from stories of place converges with the work of scholars of auto/biography like Liz Stanley, Sidonie Smith, and Julia Watson, who stress that particular institutions and social locations don't just permit personal storytelling, but can demand particular types of stories told in particular ways. As we discussed in Chapter two, certain places – the psychologist's office, the witness box, the job centre – and those listeners that people those places, "coax" particular types of narratives from people. These accounts of stories in place cut through more idealistic visions of dyadic storytelling and listening without precluding the possibility that emplaced listening might contain the potential for social change.

The socio-political view of narrative storytelling outlined above has implications for the way we understand the interpretive and socio-politico-ethical dimensions of listening. Just like storytellers, listeners are all, also, always embedded in socio-political contexts that shape the boundaries of story accessibility, listening, and interpretation. A central understanding for our work is hence that broad social and political contexts inevitably affect: (a) the accessibility of certain "kinds" of storytellers and stories in social settings; (b) listeners' willingness and inclinations to listen to certain "kinds" of stories or certain "kinds" of narrators; and (c) listeners' politically and culturally informed interpretations of stories in the event that listening even begins. The fact that digital storytelling exponents and practitioners have had to advocate for the democratising effects of digital storytelling *at all* says that some voices (for example white, male, or colonial voices) are privileged – and listened to – to such an unfair and automatic degree that others (e.g. black, indigenous, or female voices) are largely silenced and excluded in some social contexts and decision making. If we are ultimately pursuing listening as an act of social justice (which we as authors certainly are), we must also recognise that our very conceptions of social justice and marginality are shaped by larger competing meta-narratives and arrangements (see Goodman, 2011; Wilkinson & Pickett, 2009). Our understandings of and responses to the social construction of privilege, silence, and marginality hence necessarily inform how we act as practitioners who wish to promote health, well-being, and flourishing for all.

Embodied and emplaced listening

In addition to the intersubjective, social, cultural, and political "dialogues" of listening outlined above, we wish to emphasise the embodied and emplaced nature of listening. This attention to embodied and emplaced listening is, we argue, particularly relevant when discussing community and place-based health storytelling and listening but also relevant in the other contexts of listening in health and social policy and practice we cover in this book. This is because all human experience – including listening – is embodied and emplaced (see Pink, 2009). Being "embodied" means we experience and make sense of places, things, others, and ourselves via the medium of the body (Davis, 1997; Pink, 2009). Just as we might view the subject of a photo through the medium of a camera, so we must view and experience every human occurrence via the medium of our physical body and our senses. Our pre-existing embodied experience – whether it is of genetic or social origin – necessarily affects how we experience, interpret, and interact with the world around us both now and in the future. Additionally, our background and socio-economic and cultural positioning interact with the body and our subsequent health and well-being through direct physical and indirect social and cultural experiences over time (Classen, 1997, p. 401). Hence the body as a medium for experience can be seen as a highly complex, dynamic, and interpretive *filter* on listening that mediates listening just like any other medium. This filter is not only shaped by our physical wellness and sensory faculties, but also by our social and cultural experiences and the complex social settings and systems within which we are embedded throughout our lives. Bodily and sensorial experience has cultural meaning.

Just as human experience is always embodied, it is also always emplaced (Howes, 2005a; Pink, 2009). In brief, "bodies are not simply abstractions … but are embedded in the immediacies of everyday, lived experience" (Davis, 1997, p. 15). Place is central to:

> "our way of being in the world" due to the fact that we are "always emplaced … Minimally, places gather things in their midst – where 'things' connote various animate and inanimate entities. Places also gather experiences and histories, even languages and thoughts".
> (Merleau-Ponty, 1996, pp. 44 & 24, in Pink, 2009, p. 178)

Hence, place is intimately involved in producing and reproducing salient social practices and phenomena – such as storytelling, listening, history, language, thought, and identity – that shape not only our experiences of those places, but also our personal and social identities that endure across different places and times. Where we live and are "emplaced" also shapes how we see others and ourselves and how others see us (see Parry, Mathers, Laburn-Peart, Orford, & Dalton, 2007).

Deep embodied and emplaced listening

Our conceptualisation of embodied and emplaced listening hovers at the edges of time-honoured but often marginalised Indigenous and Eastern philosophical concepts of mindful embodied and emplaced experience and ways of being. Northern Australian Aboriginal educator, tribal elder, and artist Miriam Rose Ungunmerr-Baumann (2002, p. 1) for example has written about the concept of dadirri as "inner deep listening and quiet still awareness":

> [Dadirri] is something like what you call "contemplation". When I experience dadirri, I am made whole again. I can sit on the riverbank or walk through the trees; even if someone close to me has passed away, I can find my peace in this silent awareness. There is no need of words. A big part of dadirri is listening. Through the years, we have listened to our stories. They are told and sung, over and over, as the seasons go by. Today we still gather around the campfires and together we hear the sacred stories. As we grow older, we ourselves become the storytellers. We pass on to the young ones all they must know. The stories and songs sink quietly into our minds and we hold them deep inside. In the ceremonies we celebrate the awareness of our lives as sacred. The contemplative way of dadirri spreads over our whole life. It renews us and brings us peace. It makes us feel whole again … In our Aboriginal way, we learnt to listen from our earliest days. We could not live good and useful lives unless we listened. This was the normal way for us to learn – not by asking questions. We learnt by watching and listening, waiting and then acting. Our people have passed on this way of listening for over 40,000 years.
>
> (Ungunmerr-Baumann, 2002, p. 2)

The work of Ungunmerr-Baumann and internationally recognised mindfulness authors and philosophers such as Thich Nhat Hanh (Hanh, 2008) has been increasingly taken up in academic research methods (see for example, West, Stewart, Foster, & Usher, 2012); health and human services therapeutic techniques (see for example Atkinson, 1994; Delauney, 2012; Miller, Spring, Goold, Turale, & Usher, 2005; Shapiro & Carlson, 2009); and professional self-care and stress reduction practices (see for example Birnbaum, 2008; Shapiro, Astin, Bishop, & Cordova, 2005). One of the most noticeable aspects of dadirri and other contemplative, mindful, and embodied forms of listening is that it not only encourages listeners to be present and attentive for the benefit of storytellers, but also produces empirically proven benefits in terms of stress reduction, compassion for self and others, and increased quality of life *for the listeners themselves* (see Shapiro et al., 2005). Yet, while Joe Lambert has recognised the potential of mindfulness as a form of reflective practice to aid digital storytellers (Lambert, 2012, p. 127) there has not been a lot of attention to mindful, embodied, and emplaced "presence" – and the potential benefits thereof – in accounts of the way in which digital stories might be listened and responded to.

Place and health in storytelling and listening

Since the late 1980s there has been a proliferation of literature documenting the relationship between place and health (see for example Brodsky, 1996; Carpiano, Kelly, Easterbrook, & Parsons, 2011; Parry et al., 2007; Schulz & Lempert, 2004). These studies examine place-related social determinants of health (SDOH) such as natural and built environment, racism, housing, social isolation, transport, poverty, crime, and access to various types of capital (social, intellectual, economic, and so on) (Schulz & Northridge, 2004). For many health promoters, the "place-based" approach is one way to operationalise the lofty principles established in international policies and agreements such as the Ottawa Charter for Health Promotion (WHO, 1986).

Jane Farmer, Sarah-Anne Munoz, and Guinever Threlkeld (2012) have adapted social geography theory to emphasise the heterogeneity and dynamism of places that health planners and researchers often label using homogenising categories such as "peri-urban", "regional", and "remote". Farmer et al. (2012) argue instead for a dynamic conception of place and health that understands "place" as the crossing in time and space of various forces and flows (including people, economic opportunities, natural resources, social assets, politics, cultural mix, infrastructure, and history), and so as defined not only by the local but also by relatedness to other places. In keeping with this complex vision of "place", researchers in the fields of sociology of health, urban and community studies, health promotion, and social geography have developed innovative theory and methods to examine the relationship between place and health (see for example, Brodsky, 1996; Carpiano et al., 2011; Caughy, O'Campo, & Patterson, 2001).

Across a diversity of disciplines, researchers have also recognised that places and spaces do not only shape health and well-being in terms of "objective" physical or epidemiological features such as pollution or cleanliness and localised sources of infection and disease. Rather, residents' *subjective* experiences and subsequent narratives of places and spaces are also intimately interwoven with their self-rated experiences of health, well-being, and happiness (Weden et al., 2008). In their study of subjective and objective neighbourhood characteristics and adult health in the USA, Margaret Weden, Richard Carpiano, and Stephanie Robert (2008) concluded that individuals' subjective experiences and perceptions of neighbourhood quality were the most strongly linked with their self-rated health. This, along with growing attention to social and environmental determinants of health and well-being introduced in Chapter one, has reinforced the relevance of personal storytelling in place-based health promotion projects and interventions.

As a result of the growing interest in place, health, and subjective experience, we have witnessed a growing use of photovoice, digital storytelling, and social media engagement techniques in place-based research and health promotion activities internationally. Researchers and health promoters such as Joyce Yi-Frazer and colleagues (Yi-Frazer et al., 2015) and Jina Huh, Leslie Liu, Tina Neogi, Kori Inkpen, and Wanda Pratt (2014) have also combined photovoice storytelling techniques with social media platforms such as Instagram and YouTube. Others (see for example, Dennis, Gaulocher, Carpiano, & Brown, 2009; Morales-Campos, Parra-Medina, and Esparza, 2015; Sunderland, Bristed, Gudes, Boddy, & Da Silva, 2012) have mapped participant digital stories onto geographical information systems (GIS – i.e. maps of local areas) to identify "hot spots" of place-based experience that are relevant to local decision makers and health providers. A common feature of these projects is a commitment to place-based partnerships and mutual learning between researchers, health promoters, other professionals, and decision makers (see for example, Dennis et al., 2009). Digital stories generated through health and place activities are also often used for training purposes for local health and human services providers such as nurses and midwives (see for example, Hill, 2008).

At the broadest levels of place-based health promotion practice, health promoters and researchers have engaged in storytelling projects that explore the fundamental "macro" level health determinants such as climate and environment. Sherilee Harper, Victoria Edge, and Ashee Consolo Willox (2012) for example explored climate–health relationships via participatory research and digital storytelling methods within Indigenous populations of northern Canada using an EcoHealth framework. Participants created digital stories in week-long workshops with trained community members and then shared, discussed, and validated the stories with the wider community. Harper et al. (2012) concluded that the stories helped to explain climate–health relationships from various perspectives and illustrated how local people made meaning of climate and climate change events.

Notably, health researchers and health promoters often use digital storytelling as part of activities with adolescents and young people (see for example, Drew, Duncan, & Sawyer, 2010; Leung, Jun, Tseng, & Bentley, 2015; Madrigal et al., 2014; Morales-Campos et al., 2015; Willis et al., 2014; Wexler, Gubrium, Griffin, & DiFulvio, 2013); however, this is not the only demographic who have participated in health promotion-related digital storytelling and listening projects. Other international place-based health digital storytelling projects have for example explored Canadian adults' experiences and perceptions of how their community environments affect the ability to engage in physical activity (Belon, Nieuwendyk, Vallianatos, & Nykiforuk, 2014); the role that community food environments play in shaping healthy eating habits for African and Hispanic Americans with serious mental illness (Cabassa et al., 2012); and Ugandan women's experiences of obstetric fistula and the potential for "narrative medicine" practice between health practitioners and participants to co-construct stories about women's lives (Hill, 2008).

The sensorial turn

In addition to place-oriented health theory and practice, there has been a turn toward sensory embodied and emplaced research methods in place and health (see Sunderland et al., 2012). The sensory turn in social research came in response to, and partly as a criticism of, former linguistic, visual, and aural turns that saw researchers focus intensively on one mode of experience and meaning-making at the expense of others (Howes, 2005a). In contrast, sensory perspectives emphasise "the dynamic, relational (intersensory – or multimodal, multimedia) and often conflicted nature of our everyday engagement with the sensuous world" (Howes, 2005b, p. 115). Sensory approaches move beyond individual experience to identify the "cultural dimensions of corporeal [sensory] experiences and physical infrastructures ... to provide a more full-bodied understanding of social life" (Howes, 2005b, p. 115). Sensory researchers hence emphasise that sensory engagement with places and people involves diverse and complex interactions between senses (i.e. "multisensoriality") and encompasses senses that are not commonly recognised in Western cultures such as movement, progression of time, and insight (see Classen, 1993; Howes, 2005a, 2009; Kress & van Leeuwen, 1996; Pink, 2009).

A number of research and storytelling methods have since emerged that seek to share embodied and emplaced experience between storytellers and listeners either through direct shared experience of place (e.g. guided sensory walks) or through rich media representations of experience (see for example, Carpiano, 2009; Dennis et al., 2009). Our own research (see Sunderland, 2013; Sunderland et al., 2012; Sunderland, Chenoweth, Matthews, & Ellem, 2015) has drawn together the fields of place-based health and sensory ethnography with narrative inquiry and digital storytelling. These fields of inquiry and practice inform the concept of "embodied and emplaced listening" that we offer in this chapter. We now apply some of the central concepts and assumptions of our interdisciplinary theorising of embodied and emplaced listening through a case study of embodied and emplaced storytelling for health, well-being, and social justice in Logan, Australia.

Case study: Embodied and emplaced storytelling and listening with Grade 5 children

This case study has been developed from Naomi's research and community engagement activities in Logan, Australia. The case study draws on original project data, correspondence, and records as well as the researcher's own reflective narratives. The draft case study was circulated to relevant stakeholders for their review, feedback, and approval prior to publication here. The case study is also informed by a conversation conducted with Canadian-Australian narrative inquirer and early childhood specialist Marilyn Casley in 2016. Marilyn was a witness to the project as it occurred in 2010–11. This research including the conversation with Marilyn in 2016 was undertaken within ethics protocols approved by Griffith University. The case study has been anonymised in accordance with the Queensland State Education Department's research ethics requirements.

Naomi's story

In 2010–11 I had the fortune to collaborate with a local state primary school (henceforth the School), Indigenous community organisation Community Durithunga, and researchers from Griffith University's School of Human Services and Social Work and the Queensland University of Technology's School of Education to conduct a Digital Documentaries Project titled *What does it feel like to live here?* The project consisted of a three-week program of digital documentary-making workshops during school time and two field trips with Grade Five students at the School. The overarching aim of the project was to gather students' viewpoints on what makes places happy and healthy and to present them in a series of mini-documentaries to local decision makers. The *What does it feel like to live here?* project was one sub-project of a wider sensory ethnography of the Logan-Beaudesert district that I was leading at the time (see Sunderland et al., 2012). The sensory ethnography was feeding into decision making and a GIS database as part of the Logan Beaudesert Health Coalition. The project was part of an ongoing effort to identify and respond to key SDOH for local residents in the Logan-Beaudesert area. The project came after repeated research evaluation findings that community voices were not being represented or heard in the Health Coalition's ongoing planning and decision-making activities. After investigating a number of storytelling methodologies, I proposed sensory ethnography as a way that local residents could engage richly with their local environments and share rich stories of lived experiences that probably would not be recognised in other forms of statistical data for the district. Griffith University researcher Helen Bristed and I then partnered with QUT School of Education researchers including Annette Woods, Allan Luke, Kathy Mills, and John Davis-Warra who were working with the School developing digital literacies to capture the children's experiences and observations in mini-documentaries.

Listening and telling in local networks

My engagement with the School began through an invitation by my friend, colleague, and fellow musician Professor Allan Luke who had been working with the School for two years as part of the digital literacies project led by Professor Annette Woods. As I told Allan about my aims to increase residents' voices in the decision-making processes and "data" being used in the Logan Beaudesert Health Coalition he said, "hey you should come and do some stories with our kids at [the School]." Allan went on to explain to me that the students had been learning digital storytelling and documentary film-making skills in Grade four but that they had to date only made stories about relatively inconsequential things like a Roald Dahl book they had read. Allan saw our work with the Health Coalition as an opportunity for the School students to exercise and develop their rights as citizens. Allan then invited me to tell my own story about why we were doing the sensory ethnography project in Logan-Beaudesert to his broader research team at the School and to the Principal of the School. At a later date the Principal also asked me to meet with the Grade Five teachers who would be involved in the project. The teachers were keenly involved in appraising the project and linking it to their existing curriculum. The teachers also advised that it would be better to nominate selected students to participate rather than include all Grade Five students in the research. Once we had achieved research ethics approval for the project with the two participating universities and the state Education Department we began the process of engaging with the fifteen nominated students' parents to tell them about the project and invite their child to participate. We distributed letters home to parents that included an information sheet and a consent form for the parent and one for the child to read, consider, and sign. In a notable meta-oratory move, the state Education Department research ethics committee required that no school students or schools should be identifiable in research publications. This was taken up in many ways during the project including in the content of the children's stories. We had to devise a way that students could tell their stories but not have their faces shown in any of the movies which would be later shown in public.

Allan, Kathy Mills, Helen Bristed, and I also met separately with Indigenous educator, PhD researcher, and Community Durithunga representative John Davis-Warra to discuss some questions and concerns he had about people doing more research in the School and to determine what the reciprocal benefits of the research would be for the Aboriginal students at the School and their surrounding families and communities. I learnt a lot about the processes of over-researching and both overt and subtle oppression and appropriation that often accompanied "storytelling" projects involving Aboriginal and Torres Strait Islander peoples in Australia based on John's reactions and challenges to the project. His community-led advocacy, passion, and deep cultural and political knowledge revealed to me the inadequacy of my understanding of ongoing colonisation and the movement for self-determination being led by Aboriginal communities, organisations, and leaders nationally. Despite our theoretical and "best" intentions, we were heading down the track of potentially reinforcing existing oppressive and "white" privileged ways of working in this project until John stepped in as a representative of broader dialogues, opened a new conversation, and asserted both his own agency as a community leader and that of the network of elders at Community Durithunga.

Developing children's stories of embodied and emplaced experience

After several months of consultations and negotiations, the resulting *What does it feel like to live here?* project team adopted a collaborative approach to facilitating the storytelling project over three weeks of in-class time. The "hands-on" aspects of our project involved: sensitising the project team, Grade 5 teachers, and students to the concepts of SDOH; sensitising students to local Aboriginal stories about the country they walked on and the places they would visit; enhancing students' awareness of their own sensory experience of local places; teaching students how to create a mini-documentary; and teaching students to "research" how other people experienced local places. One key aim of our work with students was to help them to "turn up the senses" (Pink, 2009) so that they could make meaningful conclusions about how sensorial embodied and emplaced experience shaped their overall experiences of local places. This process of turning up the senses is done in recognition that many of us are unaware of how our sensorial experience of places shapes our overall meaning making about and responses to those places. Another key aim was to develop the students' skills in citizen research and documentary film-making. As I have mentioned, this was a core element of our QUT partners' and Community Durithunga's ongoing work with the children: to recognise their human rights as citizens and develop their capacity to observe and comment upon their own living environments. It was also at the core of the Logan Beaudesert Health Coalition's broader district-wide work in their early childhood programs.

Our first engagement with students who were nominated to participate in the *What does it feel like to live here?* project began with a yarning (talking) circle led by John Davis-Warra. John began the yarning circle with students by introducing a message stick to guide the way they would speak and listen to one another during the project. John instructed the students that whoever held the message stick could speak and the others needed to listen to that person. While standing in a small circle under a collection of gum trees in the school grounds John asked the students to think about the ways that Aboriginal people had always used their five senses to live sustainably on the country that we were all standing on. He then asked the students and other project facilitators to walk with him to a mural that had been painted in the school grounds. The mural was an Aboriginal painting that depicted cultural stories about a local lake that the students would later visit as part of a field trip for the project. John pointed out different elements of the paintings including native animals and told the students some stories about the Aboriginal country they were walking on with him. John asked the students to be like the Aboriginal custodians of the land and be mindful of what they saw, smelt, heard, tasted, and touched over the coming weeks as they moved around the local neighbourhood. So, in what felt like a very meaningful and "emplaced" introduction, the project began with the intended storytellers (student participants) *listening* to the old stories of the place and imagining what it was like for the Aboriginal people who had lived on this land for tens of thousands of years. At the end of the yarning circle John handed the message stick to a young Aboriginal student who was part of the project and instructed everyone that she would look after the message stick and that we could use it to help us tell stories and listen to one another over the coming three weeks.

The yarning circle introduction was followed up with some introductory lessons on filming that were delivered by a multimedia mentor, Josh, whom we had recruited for the project. In addition to introducing the students to the technical skills they would need to tell their stories via documentary, we also began the deliberate process of helping students to develop their embodied listening skills. We did this primarily by teaching the students to "turn up" their senses using mindfulness meditations and observation exercises in the classroom and the school grounds. One example of this was when we asked students to close their eyes and listen in the classroom. They then had to name ten things that they could hear and share it with the group. We later repeated these kinds of exercises outside the classroom in a talking circle and used the message stick to guide storytelling and listening about what people sensed and felt as they sat there together. We would ask the students to name the sensory experiences they were having and then narrate whether these experiences made them feel happy and healthy. The students then began the process of recording and representing their mindful engagement with the country using the following simple filming exercise set by the multimedia mentor Josh:

1   Film something you can see, that other people might not normally see
2   Film something natural
3   Film something made by humans
4   Film a tiny bug, animal, or insect
5   Film something that you can hear but not touch (you can see it but you can't touch it).

At the suggestion of our QUT Education team members Allan Luke and Kathy Mills, Helen Bristed and I developed a workshop exercise and handout for the students to help them develop a vocabulary for naming the embodied and emplaced experiences they were having. After we had presented students with the vocabulary worksheet we workshopped their ideas about words they would use to describe happy and healthy places and unhappy and unhealthy places. The students developed the following lists of their own terms through this exercise:

Words that the participating children used to describe happy and healthy places: safe, airy, exciting, comfortable, fun, happy, peaceful, relaxing, natural, healthy, hot, cool, fresh, loving, bright, clean, friendly, open, calm, welcoming, green, shady.

Words that the participating children used to describe unhappy and unhealthy places: smelly, unhealthy, disgusting, old, noisy, out of control, chaotic, crowded, cold, dull, rusted, uncaring, uncared for, abandoned, polluted, unsafe, and unfriendly.

These children were learning how to listen to country and place and recognise their own embodied and emplaced experiences as fundamental elements of their own stories. This listening, along with the students' later adventures in interviewing other local residents during field trips to a local lagoon and shopping centre, became the basis for their digital stories about what made them feel happy and healthy in their local environments.

A planned listening occasion

As part of my ongoing collaboration with the broader Logan Beaudesert Health Coalition I was also reporting the activities involved in the *What does it feel like to live here?* project to the district-wide network of early years childhood workers and educators. This network was facilitated by the Logan Beaudesert Health Coalition's Early Years Initiative Program and we received strong support from the Early Years Initiative's leader at that time Giselle Olive. The district-wide network was a key driving force behind Logan city being the location for the "Building a Child Friendly Community" National Conference held from November 4–5, 2011 at the Logan Entertainment Centre. The conference focused on the "growing movement of UNICEF Child Friendly Communities/Cities both internationally and nationally" (Giselle Olive, personal email communication 8/2/11) with an aim to "attract practitioners, planners and researchers keen to share and work together to build resilient communities that place children at their centre" (Giselle Olive, personal email communication 8/2/11).

We had sought sponsorship from the Early Years Initiative to pay the multimedia mentor Josh to participate in our project. As a result of this ongoing support from the Early Years Initiative and my attendance at district-wide Child Friendly Cities network meetings, the children from the *What does it feel like to live here?* project were invited to be a part of a plenary panel discussion at the UNICEF Child Friendly Cities Conference in Logan.

I include below a script that we generated with two students who acted as "hosts" for the presentation of all students' stories at the conference to give a flavour of the way that the stories were presented for listening. All participating students were invited to sit on the stage as part of a plenary panel. The two host students then introduced the other students and the documentaries and also did a mock interview with one another that was similar to the interviews they had conducted with local residents when they attended their field trips to a local shopping centre and lagoon as part of the project:

> Student 1: Hello everyone my name is [name] and this is [name]. Welcome to our part of the Building a Child Friendly Community Conference. Today we are going to show some movies that were made by Grade 5 children at [name of School]. These movies are about what we think makes places happy and healthy. We used all five of our senses to work out how we feel in different places. We also talked to people who live here to see what they think.

Student 2: Now we'd like to introduce you to the movie makers. Please say hello to: [student names are read out]. We have worked really hard to create these movies. We will show you the first four movies and then have a break. Then we will show you the final three movies. We hope you enjoy our movies. Please laugh if you want to.

First four movies are played…
Student 1: So, what do you think are some of the best things about living in Logan? [Student 2 answers]

Student 1: OK, very interesting. Now can you tell me what you think makes places happy and healthy?

Student 2: So [student 1], do you think the Logan Entertainment Centre is a happy and healthy place? Why?

Student 2: Here is my last question. Do you think school is a happy and healthy place? Why?

Student 2: Thank you everyone for being a good audience for our first four movies. We will now show you the last three movies. After that Professor Geoff [chair of the panel] will let everyone have a turn at talking.

Student 1: We hope you enjoy these movies.
Final three movies are played… Students then take questions from the audience.

After the students had presented their mini-documentaries there was time for questions from the audience members (who were, I believe, primarily adults). I think the students struggled a little bit to answer the questions that were asked of them – for example, "What do you think adults can do to make places happier for children?" The students had already answered these questions in the context of their stories and it was curious to me at the time that adult audience members wanted to ask the students the same questions "in person" and perhaps to "hear it from the horse's mouth". I remember that one audience member asked the students how they felt about showing their stories at the conference and one student answered that he felt "proud". Following the students' presentations we talked with the school Principal and the other teachers who had attended and shared what Tanja Dreher (2012) has described as a "warm glow" of shared localised storytelling and listening. On the day of the conference I don't recall anything that happened that really ruptured this warm feeling of achievement and excitement that we shared with the children and the others who had been directly involved in facilitating the project (see Figures 5.1 and 5.2).

An unplanned listening occasion

As part of our ongoing conversations about the project with the School staff and project partners, John Davis-Warra had expressed some concern that

Introduce yourself-We are researching whether our community is a healthy and happy place and we are interested in knowing how you feel about this shopping centre.

Example Questions

- Do you think this is a healthy place for you and your family or friends? Why?
- Do you like to spend time here or do you leave quickly? Why?
- What could be changed to make this a happier or healthier place?

Figure 5.1 Handout given to students to guide their community interviews for their documentaries

Interview Questions

W Do you think this is a happy place?

H Do you think this is a healthy place?

Y Do you think this is a fair place?

? Do you think this is a relaxing place?

Do you think this is a safe place?

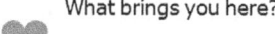 How could this be a healthier place?

W Would you like to see any changes?

H Do you think our community is healthy or unhealthy?

Y Would you come here with family or friends?

? Do you have kids who enjoy this plaza?

What brings you here?

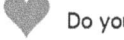 Do you come here often?

How does this place make you feel?

W How does working here impact on your family?

H Do you think it was worth taking the trees away to make this

Y shopping centre?

? Can you buy healthy food here?

Do you like to spend time here or do you leave quickly?

What could be changed to make this a happier or healthier place?

Figure 5.2 Handout summarising interview questions students had devised with facilitators prior to their field work

Aboriginal knowledges and stories might be captured and represented inappropriately or without permission in the children's documentaries. At this point I contacted Giselle Olive from the Early Years Initiative and put a halt to all plans for the children to present at the conference until we could have further talks with John and local elders at Community Durithunga. It is apparent to me now when I look back on this part of the project and on the Australian Institute for Aboriginal and Torres Strait Islander Studies (AIATSIS) principles for ethical research involving Aboriginal and Torres Strait Islander peoples (see AIATSIS, 2012) that at some times we literally don't know what we don't know and hence cannot effectively work in anti-oppressive ways. Instead, default and institutionalised dominant ways of working can and often do reinforce privileged oppressive ways of working. After some negotiation via email, John and I agreed that I would get him a USB stick with the students' final draft stories to show the elders at Community Durithunga prior to our presenting the stories at the conference in Logan. If the elders were not happy with any of the content or did not want the children to attend, we would decline the offer to participate in the conference. Hence in an unexpected but extremely valued outcome, the local elders were the very first listeners of the children's full draft digital documentary stories outside of the project facilitation team. John came back with feedback that the elders wanted to congratulate the children on their stories and that the audio was difficult to hear in places. The elders were supportive of the children taking their stories to present at the conference. Following this advice from John I contacted the conference organisers to confirm that we would be coming with the children to present their stories at the conference. My colleague Allan Luke then announced at the conference before the children showed their stories that they had the blessing of the local elders who had viewed and approved the stories. This part of our story shows once again the dynamic and complex nature of "giving voice" through digital storytelling. It also shows that in order to work in anti-oppressive ways we may need to sometimes install even more steps and acts of mediation across the storyteller's act of self-expression. This can create a complex web of consent and voice that may not initially be expected or even visible in a lot of storytelling projects.

Unexpected mediations

As I began to prepare the story of our experiences in the *What does it feel like to live here?* project for this book I remembered a story that a colleague of mine Marilyn Casley told me after the students had presented their digital stories at the UNICEF Child Friendly Cities Conference in Logan. Marilyn is an early childhood specialist and strong advocate for including children's voices in decision making at local, state, national, and international levels. In her own research Marilyn has developed techniques for adults to have meaningful and respectful conversations with children. She was presenting her work at the conference directly following the children's plenary presentation.

Marilyn said to me shortly after the conference was over that another adult attendee had vocally criticised the way the children had been included in the conference and felt that it had been exploitative of the children to ask them to sit up on the stage as part of the panel. Marilyn said that the ensuing conversation required her to respond to the delegate's vocal criticism of the children's session in order to bring the focus back to her own work. This negative feedback had surprised me at the time given that: (a) we had only received very positive feedback about the children's work and participation in the conference from the school principal, teachers, other attendees, and the children themselves; and (b) we had not heard any negative feedback whatsoever from the conference organisers or delegates. Hence this was clearly an example of an invisible and unknown mediation of meanings and response to listening by an unknown listener. We would have never been aware of it if I had not had a direct and open working relationship with Marilyn and she had not been presenting in the session directly following ours. For us, this delegate's negative reaction also brings home the need to attend to the unintended outcomes of digital storytelling and listening projects that are rarely published in academic reporting. To be honest, I think I had quite naively thought at the time that nothing bad could come from giving the children a voice, not because storytelling and listening is always beneficent but because we had put so much time and attention into putting precautions and protections in place for the children and the project partners prior to and during the entire storytelling project.

I decided to approach Marilyn to request a fuller "interview" about what she recalled about the reactions from adult delegates at the conference. Marilyn agreed to re-watch the children's documentaries before we met so that she could be reminded of their presentations at the conference and refresh her own judgements about how the children's voices were presented in their stories and listened to at the conference. When I asked Marilyn what was the most noticeable thing for her from the stories and the conference presentation, she said: "the way the community people [who were interviewed in the documentaries] took the children so seriously ... they [the adults] were really listening to the children." Marilyn's observation named yet another layer of emplaced and embodied listening and storytelling that was occurring in this project: local adult residents were listening to the children who were interviewing them. The adults' stories then literally became part of the children's stories which then became part of the story of the broader networks associated with the project and the UNESCO World Child Friendly Cities conference where the children presented.

Theorising listening

Ecosystems of listening

In her keynote address to the World Forum for Acoustic Ecology international conference in 2010, soundwalk artist Andra McCartney made simple but striking observations about the ways that listeners and listening systems overlap. In particular, McCartney explores the way that shared listening "makes a space of meaning" where different, adjacent listening "ecosystems" overlap (McCartney, 2010, n.p.). In her words:

> We could imagine the listening horizon of each listener, including the sound maker, as overlapping adjacent listening ecosystems. The act of listening to a piece makes a space of meaning where these systems overlap. Consideration of the ideas of many listeners creates a complex system of overlapping listening horizons that can provide more nuanced perspectives on the piece and its sonic meanings.
>
> (McCartney, 2010, n.p.)

For McCartney, considering the many listeners who may listen to a particular "piece" or story is inherently about connection, overlap, and complexity. She sees that each listener contains and represents an ecosystem of listening in and of themselves. She observes, further, that each listener has a listening "horizon" which represents what the listener can hear, see, feel, or understand about the piece to which they are listening at that point in time. This listening horizon is shaped by each person's listening ecosystem. We adopt McCartney's concepts of the listening ecosystem and horizon here to acknowledge that each listener represents multiple and various – simultaneous and potentially harmonious and conflicting – social roles, contexts, experiences, values, identities, and axes of power. We also think there is particular power in contemplating how listening ecosystems *overlap* and how this affects story mediation across known and unknown contexts. Every listener is mobile and dynamic within that listening ecosystem: they do not stand still or remain in the original listening environment and a person's listening horizon can extend or change over time. Hence, as McCartney observes, when listeners come together to listen to a particular story or event, we are creating a complex and unpredictable overlapping of listening ecosystems that is not limited to the time or place of listening. This applies equally to the online repositories and social media listening environments as it does to the social listening occasions – such as story project exhibitions – that were discussed in Chapter two. This was clearly the case when the students in the case study above presented their digital documentaries about place at the conference. These concepts of listening ecosystems and horizons hence significantly deepen our understandings of listening as mediation as the movement of meanings. It was also very clear in the discussion that ensued after the children's presentation during Marilyn Casley's conference presentation. The diverse listening horizons of each listener became apparent as the conference participant critiqued the way the students had been involved in the conference. The conference listening occasion also clearly created a complex space of overlapping listening ecosystems. There may be unlimited unplanned mediations of the content of the children's stories that we will never know about or be able to document as "impact" or "applications" of listening. In this case the audience members did not need to have access to the digital files from the student stories to *share their own stories* about the children and what they had seen and heard at the conference.

The unknowable nature of mediation and listening is not limited to what happens after large listening occasions such as a conference. As is evident in this case study, researchers, storytellers, and project facilitators engaged in multiple interconnected systems for place-based storytelling and listening from the moment that this project was conceived. The project itself became a temporary ecosystem of storytelling and listening that included school staff and parents, children, local health promotion and early childhood networks, and community leaders. Each act of listening then created overlaps with other ecosystems of listening such as the network of early childhood facilitators attending the conference. Each of these people, networks, and contexts had a prior history of storytelling and engagement that preceded and would exceed the duration of the project. Figure 5.3 is a basic representation of the networks of listeners who were known to be active in the listening ecosystem for the *What does it feel like to live here?* project. Each listening network is

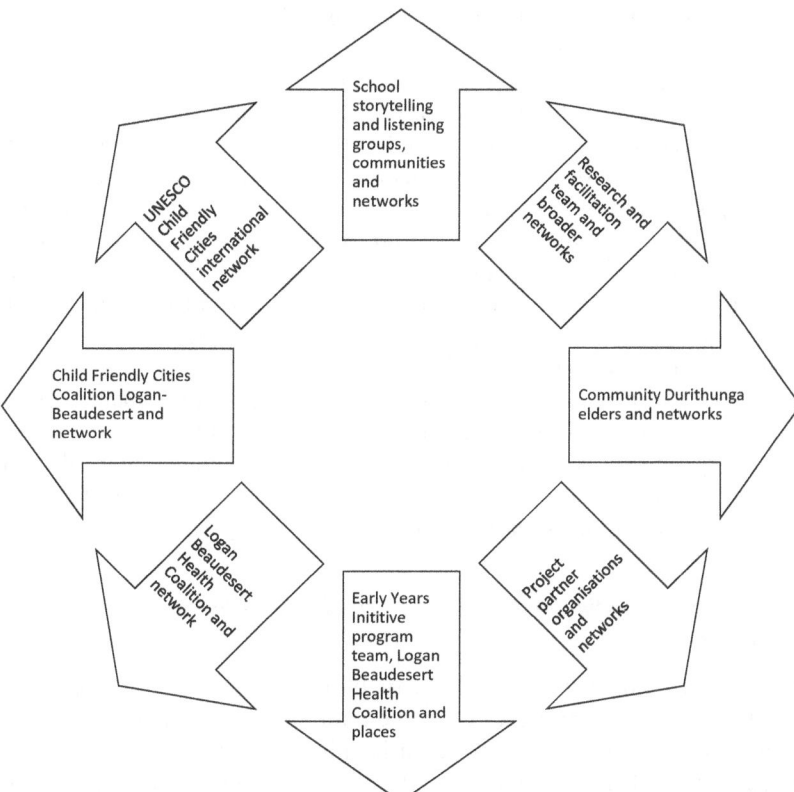

Figure 5.3 What does it feel like to live here? place-based listening ecosystem (known)

embedded in multiple and diverse listening contexts both in a social, cultural, and political sense and in the embodied and emplaced sense.

A further notable element of the case study was the degree of *deliberate* and *conscious* listening that was happening in this listening ecosystem in this health service district: multiple individuals and agencies were coming together to deliberately listen to children and attempt to effect change in children and families' lived experiences of localised SDOH. This reinforces the complexity and depth of listening and the layers of listening that can occur in place-based storytelling activities and the potential for virtually unlimited mediation and movement of meanings associated with place-based storytelling activities.

Culture and mindful listening

The facilitators' approach to listening in the above case study emphasised that all human experience is mediated via the body and thus the senses. It also acknowledged that all human experience is emplaced. Students were hence asked to listen to themselves, community leaders, each other, and country. The project facilitators assumed, further, that sensorial experience of places has potential health and well-being outcomes which were reiterated by the children in their final documentaries and also in the words they chose to describe places that were happy and healthy and unhappy and unhealthy. Following work by Pink (2009), the project facilitators also assumed, perhaps wrongly, that children and others involved in the project had been desensitised – or were never sensitised – to their sensorial experience as a matter of their embeddedness in culture. As we explored earlier in this chapter, not all cultures encourage or assume this division from sensorial experience. The dadirri concept of deep listening and connection conveyed by Ungunmerr-Baumann for example is a notable exception. In effect, an enculturated separation from or desensitisation to sensorial experience may or may not have been the case for each individual child participating in the project. Nevertheless, a starting point for both storytelling and listening was to re-sensitise participants to their embodied emplaced experience through "turning up the senses". Hence, the case study offers a reminder that both storytellers and listeners should be seen as diverse individuals with diverse cultural and individual heritages that shape even fundamental experiences of the body and place.

Communicating embodied and emplaced experience to listeners via digital artefact

Embodied and emplaced experience can be communicated in listeners in a variety of ways. For example, an embodied and emplaced listening experience might include a sensory walk through a hospital ward that features in patient stories as discussed in Chapter four. It could also include a visit to a place that was significant to storytellers such as their home or school. These types of listening experiences invite listeners to have their own experience of a social setting that will not necessarily match the storyteller's but will allow the listener to have their own lived experience of the setting that the storyteller is attempting to describe. In this way, listeners can use all of their senses to empathise, intuit, or perceive what it was like for the storyteller to experience this setting. The listener's own embodied and emplaced experience then adds an additional layer of meaning-making resources to their listening. In such cases, and if the appropriate level of self-awareness and mindfulness is present, the listener might be described as *listening with the whole body*. What happens, though, when listeners cannot or will not attend the same physical spaces to which storytellers are referring? Is deep embodied and emplaced listening still possible in these cases?

In the case study above, the storytellers' embodied and emplaced experiences of place were communicated to listeners via a digital storytelling artefact, i.e. the children's digital documentaries. The storytellers also attended a conference where their stories were shown and answered questions from the audience minimally. While many of the story listeners frequented the same geographical spaces as the children as a result of their shared focus on improving SDOH in the Logan-Beaudesert district, they did not visit the particular places the children did as a part of the listening occasions built into the project. Instead, the children went to the shared temporary context of the listeners at the World Child Friendly Cities Conference to present their stories and take questions from the audience. While we do not have project data to document how listeners experienced the content of the children's stories, we can draw on theory around media richness, sensoriality, and multimodality to further understand how multimodal texts might "deal with questions of the senses" (Pink, 2011, p. 262) and embodied and emplaced experience story content.

Extending the work of Richard Daft and Robert Lengel (1986), researchers in communication, online education, and ICT studies continue to engage media richness theory – despite some significant criticisms of this theory – to describe the way that richer media forms such as photography or video depictions have the potential to "result in higher levels of immersion or feelings of being at a ... destination" (Dinhopl & Gretzel, 2016, p. 398). Media that are "rich" in multiple modes of communication are seen to be a better "approximation" of a *specific* "real thing", i.e. *an* embodied and emplaced personal experience. Multimodality theorist Gunther Kress has argued similarly that:

> Unlike words, depictions [such as photographs or video] are full of meaning; they are always specific. So on the one hand there is a finite stock of words – vague, general, nearly empty of meaning; on the other hand there is an infinitely large potential of depictions – precise, specific, and full of meaning.
>
> (Kress, 2005, pp. 15–16)

The media richness associated with visual forms such as photography and video has been linked to communicating sensorial content and context. As

Bella Dicks, Bambo Soyinka, and Amanda Coffey articulate in their discussion of multimodal ethnography:

> Photographs allow us to see modes that are visual: colour, shape, size, position, light. What they do not show us [inherently] are modes that operate through the other senses – of touch, smell, hearing and taste – such as bodily movement, texture, three-dimensional shape, sounds.
>
> (Dicks et al., 2006, p. 88)

Yet, we also recognise that storytellers can also use single communication modes – such as vivid prose or photography – to elicit listeners' sensorial memory or imagination and a sense of "being there". While shared face-to-face or synchronous emplaced communication is sometimes regarded to be the "richest" media form due to its inclusion of all embodied and emplaced senses and communicative gestures, other theorists have argued that digital communication can result in even deeper connections between storytellers and listeners. In the early days of email and computer-mediated communication, for example, Joseph Walther (1996) found that a lack of face-to-face contact and a less rich communication medium such as email text can induce "hyper-personal" connections, intimacy, and liking between tellers and listeners that outstripped face-to-face communication. This was potentially due to the added time each party had to craft their self-representation digitally and the ability to do so without being "observed" in real time. Hence what is "visible" of the storyteller does not interfere with what is told by the storyteller. The added connection and intimacy Walther reported is also potentially due to the added time and space that listeners have to digest another's digitalised story within their own listening horizon and ecosystem.

In the case study project included in this chapter, children shot and selected footage to communicate embodied and emplaced experience that was relevant to their self-perceived health and well-being. In this case students were using a rich media form to deliberately communicate embodied and emplaced experience and were inviting listeners to co-experience that place through the digital mini-documentary. In this way the children – and any other storytellers for that matter – can invoke the multimodal, artistic, and evocative elements of story and representation to induce listeners' embodied sensorial memory or imagination. All human experience is multisensorial: we are used to "listening" with our whole bodies. Hence we can use imagination and prior experience to listen to personal stories with our whole body. Although the listeners may or may not ever frequent the same places that the children did when making their films, listeners have the potential to carry the children's stories as part of their own listening horizon and ecosystem. If a listener ever did visit the same places that the children did, they may remember and revisit their own account of the children's stories voluntarily or involuntarily based on the stimulus of their own current lived experience. Or, listeners may *apply* the children's stories to any similar or different environment as part of their dynamic movement through the world. A listener could take the lessons that they learned from the children's stories – such as a favouring for quiet, green, warm, and friendly spaces – and apply them to new contexts such as designing children's play space in a community centre or clinic. This, as we discussed in Chapter one, is listening as mediation: the movement of meanings across contexts and into increasingly durable materialities (Iedema, 2000). Whether or not listeners actually do this – and hence incite visible and sustainable social change – is another matter.

Take-aways for practitioners

- All listening is fundamentally embodied and emplaced. This is unavoidable.
- All human experience is multisensorial: we listen with our whole bodies all of the time. This is our normal way of engaging with the world whether we choose to do it and are aware of it or not.
- All listening occurs within wider socio-political and cultural contexts which can be produced, reproduced, and challenged through the conduct of storytelling and listening activities.
- Deep embodied and emplaced listening is encouraged as a daily normal practice in many marginalised cultures. It is not routinely encouraged in Westernised cultures that promote separation from nature and busy, hectic lifestyles.
- Deep embodied and emplaced listening can occur when listeners mindfully engage with a place that is important to a storyteller such as a local nature reserve or hospital ward. It can also occur when listeners cannot share the same place with a storyteller but mindfully engage with digital story artefacts and allow remembered or imagined embodied and emplaced experience to supplement meaning making. Deep embodied and emplaced listening is hence arguably a deeper form of empathetic listening.
- Sensorial experience of place – and its effects on health and well-being – is often overlooked. Attention to embodied and emplaced experience provides a richer palette of meaning-making resources for listeners to make sense of and respond to story content.

Conclusion

In this chapter we have introduced a number of distinct features of storytelling and listening in community and place-based health and social care policy and practice. We argue that embodied and emplaced listening potentially creates a more deeply "contextualised" view of storytellers and stories among listeners. It can also create opportunities for listeners to directly sense, intuit, feel, see, hear, touch, taste, or smell what the storyteller might have experienced and portrayed in their story. In essence, conscious and mindful embodied and emplaced listening has the potential to occur through the listener's "whole" body and self. This is relevant for understanding place as a social determinant of health, developing listening approaches and skills, and potentially in the design of places and spaces linked to health and well-being.

References

AIATSIS (2012). *Guidelines for Ethical Research in Australian Indigenous Studies.* Retrieved from http://aiatsis.gov.au/sites/default/files/docs/research-and-guides/ethics/GERAIS.pdf

Atkinson, J. (1994). Recreating the circle with WE AL-LI: A program for healing, sharing and regeneration. *Aboriginal and Islander Health Worker Journal, 18*(6), 8–13.

Bavelas, J. B., Coates, L., & Johnson, T. (2000). Listeners as co-narrators. *Journal of Personality and Social Psychology, 79*(6), 941–952.

Beck, C. S. (2005). Becoming the story: Narratives as collaborative, social enactments of individual, relational, and public identities. In L. M. Harter, P. M. Japp, & C. S. Beck (Eds.), *Narratives, Health and Healing: Communication Theory, Research, and Practice* (pp. 61–82). Mahwah, NJ: Lawrence Erlbaum Associates.

Belon, A. P., Nieuwendyk, L. M., Vallianatos, H., & Nykiforuk, C. I. (2014). How community environment shapes physical activity: Perceptions revealed through the PhotoVoice method. *Social Science & Medicine, 116*, 10–21.

Birnbaum, L. (2008). The use of mindfulness training to create an 'accompanying place' for social work students. *Social Work Education, 27*(8), 837–852.

Brodsky, A. E. (1996). Resilient single mothers in risky neighborhoods: Negative psychological sense of community. *Journal of Community Psychology, 24*(4), 347–363.

Cabassa, L. J., Parcesepe, A., Nicasio, A., Baxter, E., Tsemberis, S., & Lewis-Fernández, R. (2012). Health and wellness photovoice project engaging consumers with serious mental illness in health care interventions. *Qualitative Health Research, 20*(10), 1–13. doi:10.1177/1049732312470872.

Carpiano, R., (2009). Come take a walk with me: The 'go-along' interview as a novel method for studying the implications of place for health and well-being. *Health and Place, 15*(1), 263–272.

Carpiano, R. M., Kelly, B. C., Easterbrook, A., & Parsons, J. T. (2011). Community and drug use among gay men: The role of neighborhoods and networks. *Journal of Health & Social Behavior, 52*(1), 74–90.

Caughy, M. O., O'Campo, P. J., & Patterson, J. (2001). A brief observational measure for urban neighborhoods. *Health & Place, 7*(3), 225–236.

Clandinin, D. J., & Connelly, F. M. (2000). *Narrative Inquiry: Experience and Story in Qualitative Research.* San Francisco, CA: Jossey-Bass.

Classen, C. (1993). *Worlds of Sense: Exploring the Senses in History and across Culture.* London: Routledge.

Classen, C. (1997). Foundations for an anthropology of the senses . *International Social Science Journal, 49*(153), 401–412.

Connelly, F. M., & Clandinin, D. J. (1990). Stories of experience and narrative inquiry. *Educational Researcher, 19*(5), 2–14.

Daft, R., & Lengel, R. (1986). Organizational information requirements, media richness and structural design. *Management Science, 32*(5), 554–571.

Davis, K. (1997). Embodying theory: Beyond modernist and postmodernist readings of the body. In K. Davis (Ed.), *Embodied Practices: Feminist Perspectives on the Body* (pp. 2–26). London: Sage.

Delauney, T. (2012). Fractured culture: Educare as a healing approach to indigenous trauma. *International Journal of Science in Society, 4*(1), 53–62.

Dennis, S. F., Gaulocher, S., Carpiano, R. M., & Brown, D. (2009). Participatory photo mapping (PPM): Exploring an integrated method for health and place research with young people. *Health & Place, 15*(2), 466–473.

Dicks, B., Soyinka, B., & Coffey, A. (2006). Multimodal ethnography. *Qualitative Research, 6*(1), 77–96.

Dinhopl, A., & Gretzel, U. (2016). Conceptualizing tourist videography. *Information Technology & Tourism, 15*(4), 395–410.

Dreher, T. (2012). A partial promise of voice: Digital storytelling and the limit of listening. *Media International Australia, 142*(1), 157–166.

Drew, S. E., Duncan, R. E., & Sawyer, S. M. (2010). Visual storytelling: A beneficial but challenging method for health research with young people. *Qualitative Health Research, 20*(12), 1677–1688.

Farmer, J., Munoz, S. A., & Threlkeld, G. (2012). Theory in rural health. *Australian Journal of Rural Health, 20*(4), 185–189. doi:10.1111/j.1440-1584.2012.01286.x

Goodman, D. J. (2011). *Promoting Diversity and Social Justice: Educating People from Privileged Groups.* London: Routledge.

Hanh, T. N. (2008). *The Miracle of Mindfulness: The Classic Guide to Meditation by the World's Most Revered Master.* North Sydney: Random House.

Harper, S. L., Edge, V. L., & Willox, A. C. (2012). 'Changing climate, changing health, changing stories' profile: Using an EcoHealth approach to explore impacts of climate change on Inuit health. *EcoHealth, 9*(1), 89–101.

Hill, A. L. (2008). 'Learn from my story': A participatory media initiative for Ugandan women affected by obstetric fistula. *Agenda, 22*(77), 48–60.

Howes, D. (2005a). Architecture of the senses. In M. Zardini (Ed.), *Sense of the City: An Alternate Approach to Urbanism* (pp. 322–331). Montreal: Canadian Centre for Architecture and Lars Müller Publishers.

Howes, D. (2005b). Charting the sensorial revolution. *Senses & Society, 1*(1), 113–128.

Howes, D. (Ed.) (2009). *The Sixth Sense Reader.* Oxford: Berg.

Huh, J., Liu, L. S., Neogi, T., Inkpen, K., & Pratt, W. (2014). Health vlogs as social support for chronic illness management. *ACM Transactions on Computer-Human Interaction (TOCHI), 21*(4), 23–31.

Iedema, R. (2000). Bureaucratic planning and resemiotisation. In E. Ventola (Ed.), *Discourse and Community. Doing Functional Linguistics* (pp. 47–70). Tubingen: Narr Verlag.

Kim, J. H. (2016). *Understanding Narrative Inquiry: The Crafting and Analysis of Stories as Research.* Los Angeles, CA: Sage.

Kress, G. (2005). Gains and losses: New forms of texts, knowledge, and learning. *Computers and Composition, 22*(1), 5–22.

Kress, G., & van Leeuwen, T. (1996). *Reading Images: The Grammar of Visual Design.* London: Routledge.

Krug, E. G., Mercy, J. A., Dahlberg, L. L., & Zwi, A. B. (2002). The world report on violence and health. *The Lancet, 360*(9339), 1083–1088.

Lambert, J. (2012). *Digital Storytelling: Capturing Lives, Creating Community.* London: Routledge.

Langellier, K. M. (1989). Personal narratives: Perspectives on theory and research. *Text and Performance Quarterly, 9*(4), 243–276.

Langellier, K. (2011). *Storytelling in Daily Life: Performing Narrative.* Philadelphia, PA: Temple University Press.

Leung, M. M., Jun, J., Tseng, A., & Bentley, M. (2015). 'Picture me healthy': A pilot study using photovoice to explore health perceptions among migrant youth in Beijing, China. *Global Health Promotion*. doi: 10.1177/1757975915594126.

McCartney, A. (2010, June). Ethical questions about working with soundscapes. Soundwalking interactions. Keynote presented at WFAE international conference Ideologies and Ethics in the Uses and Abuses of Sound, Koli, Finland.

Madrigal, D., Salvatore, A., Casillas, G., Casillas, C., Vera, I., Eskenazi, B., & Minkler, M. (2014). Health in my community: Conducting and evaluating PhotoVoice as a tool to promote environmental health and leadership among Latino/a youth. *Progress in Community Health Partnerships: Research, Education, and Action*, *8*(3), 317–329.

Miller, M., Spring, L., Goold, S., Turale, S., & Usher, K. (2005). *Dadirri: A Nursing Guide to Improving Indigenous Health. Report from the Indigenous Nursing Education Working Group.* Canberra: Office of Aboriginal and Torres Strait Islander Health.

Morales-Campos, D. Y., Parra-Medina, D., & Esparza, L. A. (2015). Picture this! Using participatory photo mapping with Hispanic girls in a community-based participatory research project. *Family & Community Health*, *38*(1), 44–54.

Parry, J., Mathers, J., Laburn-Peart, C., Orford, J., & Dalton, S. (2007). Improving health in deprived communities: What can residents teach us? *Critical Public Health, 17*(2), 123–136. doi: 10.1080/09581590601045253

Pink, S. (2009). *Doing Sensory Ethnography.* Los Angeles, CA: Sage.

Pink, S. (2011). Multimodality, multisensoriality and ethnographic knowing: Social semiotics and the phenomenology of perception. *Qualitative Research*, *11*(3), 261–276.

Reading, C. L., & Wien, F. (2009). *Health Inequalities and the Social Determinants of Aboriginal Peoples' Health.* Prince George: National Collaborating Centre for Aboriginal Health.

Schulz, A., & Lempert, L. (2004). Being part of the world: Detroit women's perceptions of health and social environment. *Journal of Contemporary Ethnography*, *33*(4), 437–465.

Schulz, A., & Northridge, M. E. (2004). Social determinants of health: Implications for environmental health promotion. *Health Education & Behavior*, *31*(4), 455–471.

Shapiro, S. L., Astin, J. A., Bishop, S. R., & Cordova, M. (2005). Mindfulness-based stress reduction for health care professionals: Results from a randomized trial. *International Journal of Stress Management*, *12*(2), 164–176.

Shapiro, S. L., & Carlson, L. E. (2009). *The Art and Science of Mindfulness: Integrating Mindfulness into Psychology and the Helping Professions.* London: American Psychological Association.

Sunderland, N. (2013). Outside the cage: Exploring everyday interactions between government workers and residents in a place-based health initiative. *Advances in Applied Sociology*, *3*(1), 61–68.

Sunderland, N., Bristed, H., Gudes, O., Boddy, J., & Da Silva, M. (2012). What does it feel like to live here? Exploring sensory ethnography as a collaborative methodology for investigating social determinants of health in place. *Health & Place*, *18*(5), 1056–1067.

Sunderland, N., Chenoweth, L., Matthews, N., & Ellem, K. (2015). 1000 Voices: Reflective online multimodal narrative inquiry as a research methodology for disability research. *Qualitative Social Work*, *14*(1), 48–64. doi: 1473325014523818.

Ungunmerr-Baumann, M. R. (2002). *Dadirri: Inner Deep Listening and Quiet Still Awareness* [educational brochure]. Retrieved from http://nextwave.org.au/wp-content/uploads/Dadirri-Inner-Deep-Listening-M-R-Ungunmerr-Bauman-Refl.pdf

Walther, J. B. (1996). Computer-mediated communication: Impersonal, interpersonal, and hyperpersonal interaction. *Communication Research, 23*(1), 3–43.

Weden, M. M., Carpiano, R. M., & Robert, S. A. (2008). Subjective and objective neighborhood characteristics and adult health. *Social Science & Medicine, 66*(6), 1256–1270.

West, R., Stewart, L., Foster, K., & Usher, K. (2012). Through a critical lens. Indigenist research and the Dadirri method. *Qualitative Health Research, 22*(11), 1582–1590.

Wexler, L., Gubrium, A., Griffin, M., & DiFulvio, G. (2013). Promoting positive youth development and highlighting reasons for living in Northwest Alaska through digital storytelling. *Health Promotion Practice, 14*(4), 617–623.

WHO (1986). *Ottawa Charter for Health Promotion.* Retrieved from http://www.who. int/healthpromotion/conferences/previous/ottawa/en/

Wilkinson, R., & Pickett, K. (2009). *The Spirit Level: Why Greater Equality Makes Societies Stronger.* New York: Bloomsbury Press.

Wilkinson, R. G., & Marmot, M. G. (2003). *Social Determinants of Health: The Solid Facts.* Geneva: WHO.

Willis, N., Frewin, L., Miller, A., Dziwa, C., Mavhu, W., & Cowan, F. (2014). "My story" – HIV positive adolescents tell their story through film. *Children and Youth Services Review, 45*, 129–136.

Yi-Frazer, J. P., Cochrane, K., Mitrovich, C., Pascual, M., Buscaino, E., Eaton, L., Panlasigui, N., Clopp, B., & Malik, F. (2015). Using Instagram as a modified application of PhotoVoice for storytelling and sharing in adolescents with type 1 diabetes. *Qualitative Health Research, 25*(10), 1372–1382.

6 Are policymakers listening?

In this chapter we make our final move away from the one-to-one exchange between storytellers and listener that has been at the centre of most under-standings of listening, and turn to the way personal digital stories might be used in the formation of national and international policy. As well as review-ing the existing literature on digital storytelling in policymaking contexts, we focus our discussion on two case studies: the Australian *National Disability Insurance Scheme* (NDIS) and Handicap International's *Ban Advocates* initiative, to shed more light onto how digital stories are and can be used in policymaking. Research in this arena is challenging thanks to the opaque nature of much decision making in local, state, national, and international policymaking settings. In this chapter we discuss the known outcomes and uses of digital stories in policymaking reported in existing academic literature. We then compare what is reported in the academic literature with our own case studies and theorise current practice in terms of its significance for listening. Our focus as we delve further into our case studies will be an exploration of the practices deployed by advocates and policymakers when drawing on digital storytelling as a resource for policymaking.

How and why are people using digital stories in policymaking and to what effect?

There are strong historical links between testimonial practices such as digital storytelling and liberation movements such as feminism, resistance against dic-tatorship, holocaust testimony, and civil rights movements (see for example, Funkenstein, 1993; Sillato, 2008). Such projects have aimed to help victims of trauma and torture, young people, elderly people, people who are unemployed, or who experience disability summarise, capture, and share meaningful life experiences "with a view to effecting social change that will improve their future experiences" (Lundby, 2008, p. 363). Yet the processes by which this storytelling might help change the policymaking settings which direct public investment and shape the quality of life for these people have rarely been examined in any detail.

As Helga Lénárt-Cheng and Darija Walker (2011) have pointed out, while listening to and sharing digital stories are foregrounded in the *rationales* of some projects, there are often very few concrete strategies in place to achieve policy influence. Instead, the ultimate outcomes of digital storytelling are often presented as storytelling being an enactment of democracy in itself. As Lénárt-Cheng and Walker note, for some digital storytelling projects "the act of sharing functions ... not as a means to achieve democracy, but as an actual act of democracy. According to these activists, the dialogue constituted by life story-sharing already equals activism" (Lénárt-Cheng & Walker, 2011, p. 150). While we agree at least in sentiment with this view that making diverse stories available is often an act of resistance and celebration of plurality in itself, we need to go much further if we are to answer the question: are policymakers listening?

Digital storytelling practitioners' commitments to promoting authentic, relatively unmediated individual voice often exist in tension with the very evident processes of mediation, remediation, and recontextualisation involved in using life narratives in policymaking settings. This tension has often been skirted around in academic and project-related writing about digital storytelling by including a gesture towards the policy impacts of storytelling – a "leap of faith" – rather than a careful mapping of how such impacts might play out in practice. What we mean by referring to a "leap of faith" is that at times "influencing policy" or "influencing policymakers" becomes a throwaway line about project outcomes rather than a budgeted, practical, and strategic plan for ally work, advocacy, and activism. In these cases there is no doubt a genuine wish that social justice will occur but arguably little real active and ongoing investment in or understanding of how that might happen. The NDIS in Australia – which we consider below – was an example of a consultation process where disability storytellers and advocates were arguably asked to take a leap of faith in submitting stories for policymaking purposes. As we discuss in the NDIS case study, in many cases policymaking that draws on digital stories or other forms of autobiographical narrative takes place in a "black box": narratives are submitted but outsiders cannot see what is done with or to those stories in the processes of making policy.

In our own work on the *1000 Voices* disability life stories project we have experienced this "black box" effect which makes it difficult to discern exactly how, or indeed whether, digital stories are being used "behind closed doors" in policymaking contexts. For many digital storytelling advocates it is possible to witness, and potentially influence, the "inputs" of policymaking through the creation and contribution of digital stories or the generation of discussion papers. What happens within the black box of actual decision making often remains a mystery (see Flitcroft, Gillespie, Salkeld, Carter, & Trevena, 2011). It might appear possible, in a policy context, to identify whether listening and response to digital stories are taking place by simply comparing the life stories contributed to public consultation exercises to the policies that emerge from these in order to assess whether or how listening is taking place. Yet, as work around public participation in policymaking more generally has pointed out, things are not so simple. It is widely agreed that decision-making processes around policy are not linear or based primarily on rational evaluation of available evidence and are shaped more by the "exigencies of the moment" (Flitcroft et al., 2011, p. 1043; see also Nutbeam & Boxall, 2008). In addition, as Mavis Jones and Edna Einsiedel (2011) argue, rather than looking for immediate outcomes from public participation, change might be better imagined in terms of incremental "institutional learning" (p. 656).

Mapping of existing literature

In this section we draw on existing academic literature to further address two questions: (a) whether policymakers are listening at all; and (b) whether policymakers are only listening in and on their own terms. The relatively sparse published research on digital storytelling and policymaking offers some insights into how and why people are using digital stories in policymaking and to what effect. It also offers some evaluation of the "impact" of digital storytelling on listeners through different levels of social change and action. Table 6.1 summarises existing studies of digital storytelling projects using an adapted program logic model format. The program logic model in its full form is often used in health, human services, and education research evaluations (see Hernandez, 2000) to identify the context and assumptions underpinning an "intervention" and then track desired deliverables and short-, medium-, and long-term or "ultimate" outcomes. In its full form, the program logic model helps organisations and coalitions to identify the implicit or explicit theory of change underpinning their work and to ensure that their stated aims are being achieved in terms of deliverables and outcomes.

We have used an adapted program logic format in Table 6.1 to map out information from existing published studies in order to tease out the known outcomes that have arisen from digital storytelling projects or activities that have had a specific aim to influence policy and decision makers. Table 6.1 reviews all articles returned via a Summon peer-reviewed journal database in January 2014 using the search terms "digital story" and "policy". Only those articles that were substantially focused on digital storytelling and policymaking processes were selected for full review here. The range of deliverables or outputs from digital storytelling projects and activities included in Table 6.1 reflect the intersectional use of digital stories with other digital media and offline advocacy and engagement work. Our primary adaptation to Hernandez's logic model template was to remove columns associated with "inputs" and "assumptions" given that we are focused on the outcomes of storytelling in this chapter and book more broadly. We have also added the terms individual, micro, meso, and macro to Hernandez's existing categories of short-, medium-, and long-term outcomes to link back to the SDOH framework outlined in Chapter one and the diverse contexts covered in earlier chapters of this book. Ultimate outcomes according to program logic methodology are the larger more sustainable

Table 6.1 Examples of policy and social change/justice outcomes from digital storytelling (from existing literature)

Program, Organisation, Source	Situation or context What were the needs? Why were people using digital stories?	Outputs What did people produce or do?	Reported outcomes Short term Individual and micro (interpersonal)	Reported outcomes Medium term Meso (community)	Reported outcomes Ultimate Macro (societal)
Silence Speaks Program, Center for Digital Storytelling (USA) Africa storytelling projects on HIV/AIDs and labour migration (Polk, 2010)	• Activist organising and education • Technique for increasing understanding of social stigmas such as people living with AIDS/HIV • As a way for victims of trauma and violence to speak out about their experiences • Highlighting the issues and consequences of labour migration	• HIV/AIDs digital stories • Discussion guides • Story screenings across southern Africa • DVD of labour migrant stories • Facilitator's guide to raise awareness	• Offer "testimonials about survival" (n.p.) • Facilitate local discussions about the content covered in the digital stories • Encouraging others to be tested and treated for HIV/AIDS	• Challenged "stereotyped representations of men, women, and gender-based violence in popular media" (n.p.) • Challenged "misperceptions about men and masculinity and offer examples of the role both men and women play in confronting forms of injustice" (n.p.) • "Educating local communities, training service providers, inspiring policymakers" (n.p.) • "Making these stories public online, makes them available to human rights and labor organizations all over the world as documented real-life data" (n.p.)	• Potential to reinforce cultural oppression, e.g. through Westernised storytelling model being used in Africa

Program, Organisation, Source	Situation or context What were the needs? Why were people using digital stories?	Outputs What did people produce or do?	Reported outcomes Short term Individual and micro (interpersonal)	Reported outcomes Medium term Meso (community)	Reported outcomes Ultimate Macro (societal)
	"sustainable social change ... a lasting process of empowerment and transformation that aids in the reduction of poverty and makes possible greater social equality and the larger fulfillment of human potential" (np)			• "Creates a space for the oppressed to speak on their own terms and to be potentially heard by others like themselves in similar situations around the world, thus aiding in the creation of [virtual] communities" (n.p.) • Potential to reinforce expert-led model of media production	
Information Cultural Exchange Western Sydney, Australia Public screenings of digital stories (Dreher, 2012)	• "Facilitating cultural production" (p. 160) • Providing "opportunities for participants to have their voices' heard", e.g. through public screenings (p. 160) • Providing opportunity for participants to showcase their work • Inviting respect and recognition for storytellers • Giving storytellers a voice	• Collection of "mini-films" • Public launch event • Invited local councillors, and state and federal members of parliament to attend launch • Inviting artists and industry professionals to attend the launch	• "Noticeable 'buzz' and 'feel-good mood'" • Infectious atmosphere of celebration (p. 161) • "Digital storytellers are celebrated for 'speaking up' and claiming 'voice'" (p. 163)	• "A lack of institutional commitments to political listening" by decision makers who attended (p. 158) • Positioning storytellers as "(cultural) citizens" (p. 160) • Positioning storytellers as "cultural artists" (p. 161) • Intercommunal listening (Mowbray, 2010, in Dreher, 2012, p. 161) • Intergenerational listening (Salazar, 2010; Lee-Shoy & Dreher, 2009 in Dreher, 2012, p. 161)	• Limited effect of stories on audiences outside of local region • "Little opportunity to explore the ways in which politicised voices might make a difference" (p. 163)

Program, Organisation, Source	Situation or context What were the needs? Why were people using digital stories?	Outputs What did people produce or do?	Reported outcomes Short term Individual and micro (interpersonal)	Reported outcomes Medium term Meso (community)	Reported outcomes Ultimate Macro (societal)
				• Intergenerational listening (Salazar, 2010; Lee-Shoy & Dreher, 2009 in Dreher, 2012, p. 161) • Stories primarily circulated in "community sector" rather than via broadcast media (p. 161) • Concerns from storytellers and facilitators that the stories are not travelling far enough away from the local storytelling context in terms of who is listening to them (p. 162) • Storyteller concerns that decision makers need to hear their stories but are not hearing them (p. 162) • Even where digital storytelling is used with the specific purpose of community, "events do not foreground debate or politics or issues or advocacy in the conventional sense" (p. 163)	

Program, Organisation, Source	Situation or context What were the needs? Why were people using digital stories?	Outputs What did people produce or do?	Reported outcomes Short term Individual and micro (interpersonal)	Reported outcomes Medium term Meso (community)	Reported outcomes Ultimate Macro (societal)
				• Limited effect of stories on audience members who are "resistant to hearing them" (interviewee report in Dreher, 2012, p. 161) • "The atmosphere of celebration … seemed to work against overtly political forms of listening or engagement with digital stories" (p. 162) • "Issues behind more politicised stories are unlikely to be meaningfully or productively discussed" (p. 163)	
Reach Out! (www.reachout.com.au) and ActNow (www.actnow.com.au) National projects	Provide "information, support and resources to improve young people's understanding of mental health issues, and help them to develop resilience, increase coping skills, and facilitate help-seeking behaviour" (p. 532)	"Utilise a range of Web-based (public forums, digital stories and online games) and mobile applications (podcasts and Short Message Service (SMS) campaigns) to engage with young people" (p. 532)	• Young people were able to seek information about issues they were concerned about • Young people received training	"The internet was seen as a vehicle for achieving multiple goals: doing something about the issues, meeting new people, generating networks, and gaining experience 'for the future'. It was also perceived as a very important tool for identifying causes, learning more, responding to issues, and integrating participation into everyday life" (p. 534)	• "Shift away from dutiful citizens to actualising citizens" (Bennett, 2007, in Collin, 2008, p. 535) • Participants reported that the existing power and influence of government institutions were not disrupted through these programs

Program, Organisation, Source	Situation or context What were the needs? Why were people using digital stories?	Outputs What did people produce or do?	Reported outcomes Short term Individual and micro (interpersonal)	Reported outcomes Medium term Meso (community)	Reported outcomes Ultimate Macro (societal)
Inspire Foundation, Australia (Collin, 2008)	• Provide young people with "opportunities to find out more about their world and take action on the issues they care about" • Provide young people with access to "information, organisations, networks and other people, as well as tools for taking action" (p. 532) • Enrol young people as "youth ambassadors" to engage in online public participation activities and training	• "Formal mechanisms are managed by Inspire staff, whereas informal mechanisms are driven by young people" (p. 532)	• Participants retained "perception that governments and politicians were old, exclusive and hierarchical" (p. 535)	• Young people were able to "control how and when they are involved" in public participation activities (p. 534) • "Develop a sense of connectedness, meaningfulness and ownership" (p. 534) • Provides young people with a "forum to act on issues that they care about, while being relevant to their lifestyles" (p. 534) • Employment generation for three participants in youth-service organisations • Participating young people saw the Internet as a vehicle for self-expression, political agency, and influence outside of formal government initiatives, e.g. via non-government organisations (NGOs)	• "Youth participation policies in government are associated with being spoken at, exclusive or elitist processes, and lack of control, but also that the use of the internet to deliver these policies perpetuates elitism" • "Non-government, youth-led and interest-based communities and organisations' use of the internet was considered to be open and democratic, resisting the tendency to control or manage forms of participation" (p. 536)

Program, Organisation, Source	Situation or context What were the needs? Why were people using digital stories?	Outputs What did people produce or do?	Reported outcomes Short term Individual and micro (interpersonal)	Reported outcomes Medium term Meso (community)	Reported outcomes Ultimate Macro (societal)
				• Participants saw "government use of the internet as an extension of the control that governments exercise over off-line youth participation" (p. 535) • Participating "NGOs were seen … as new, inclusive and discursive. Interviewees saw themselves as playing a valuable, legitimate role in the Inspire Foundation, rather than as 'programme recipients'" (p. 535) • Youth participants took on advocacy and activist roles in other online and offline projects • Internet-based participation overcame obstacles associated with geographical distance, mental health issues, and dominant conceptions of what a "good" and "active" citizen is (p. 537) • Young people felt forced to participate on the government's terms and within government templates and time frames (p. 535)	• "Despite the potential for participation policies and the internet to mitigate elitism and inequality in youth participation, there is little evidence to suggest that this is occurring in practice" (p. 537) • "The internet served to mobilise new forms of participation among young people who do not consider themselves to be 'politically active'" (p. 537)

Program, Organisation, Source	Situation or context What were the needs? Why were people using digital stories?	Outputs What did people produce or do?	Reported outcomes Short term Individual and micro (interpersonal)	Reported outcomes Medium term Meso (community)	Reported outcomes Ultimate Macro (societal)
Participate International network Participatory research to influence development policy (Shahrokh & Wheeler, 2014)	• To influence global goals for development through participatory research (p. 9) • To promote participation, development, democracy, social justice, gender equality, sustainability, and social inclusion (p. 7) • The aims of the Participate network are to: • Bring perspectives of those in poverty into decision-making processes • Embed participatory research in global policymaking • Use research with the poorest as the basis for advocacy with decision makers	• International network of existing NGOs working with marginalised peoples • Participatory video • Community radio, digital storytelling with creative writing, storyboarding, and role-playing • Ground Level Panels (GLPs) "used to contrast the closed space of United Nations (UN) High Level Panel (HLP)" • Film documentary set in eight countries	• "The power of visuals, stories and the personal for communication, and the importance of relationships" (p. 5) • Participants connect with others in similar situations, aggregate knowledge, build "more complete understandings of situations", share strategies for local action, build coalitions for wider political action (p. 14) "Participants come to recognise, value and act upon their own inherent knowledge, skills, experiences – their 'power within'" (VeneKlasen & Miller, 2007, p. 14)	• Lessons on "what disturbingly hasn't worked is a stark challenge for the future" (p. 5) • "Participatory processes create a distinctive form of knowledge … [which] challenges and changes power relations" (p. 14) • Transformed research processes that challenge dominant ways of conceiving of knowledge and research process • Exploded "preconceptions and biases of researchers and their organisations" (p. 14) • "New relationships are formed, new communities within communities organise, elements of the fragmented community cohere to address a common cause" (p. 14)	• Transformed power relations between researchers and research participants (people who experience marginalisation) • Persisting "extraordinary contrast between the uniformity of [elite privileged] policy-makers and the diversity of those who are marginalised" (p. 5) • "Participatory methodologies do not have to be standardised to be effective" (p. 5)

Program, Organisation, Source	Situation or context What were the needs? Why were people using digital stories?	Outputs What did people produce or do?	Reported outcomes Short term Individual and micro (interpersonal)	Reported outcomes Medium term Meso (community)	Reported outcomes Ultimate Macro (societal)
	• "Ensure that marginalised people have a central role in holding decision makers to account in the post-2015 process Generate knowledge, understanding, and relationships for the global public good • "To collapse the distance between every day experiences of marginalisation and global decision-making" (p. 10) • "Move policy-makers beyond a purely rational assessment of the research into a space where they built more connected relationships with people living in poverty and marginalisation" (p. 11)	• Exhibition in New York • 18 studies • Field-tested new methodological tools • Global synthesis report which has had recognisable influence on the post-2015 debate Engagement in meetings of the UN Post-2015 High Level Panel of Eminent Persons (HLP) • Website, blog, and Twitter account Written policy briefings • Visiting fellowships • Workshops	• "27 members of the UN High Level Panel for [development] planning were each given the opportunity of a brief immersion living with marginalised people. Not a single one took it up" (p. 5)	• Increased "understanding of where there is room to maneuver and to act to make change, and also to understand the power in the system and its contribution to their [people who experience oppression] marginalisation" (p. 16) • "Even in processes such as digital storytelling (DST) 8 where the output may be a single individual's narrative, the space in which that narrative is created is one of shared experience and collective analysis" (p. 16) • "A deeper grasp of the whole of the situation, and provokes new questions about the sources of problems and reveals capacities for action within the community to respond to the pressing concerns which have been raised" (p. 16)	• "The grounded, narrative nature of participatory outputs enable policy-makers to understand more specifically the limitations and gaps in existing policy and practice. Through participatory research, the counter-hegemonic knowledge of the poor and marginal can enter physically and politically inaccessible spaces via research conduits" (p. 14) • "The recovery of ideas and worldviews that have been undermined by policy, media and education systems which stigmatise and belittle the knowledge that people inherently have as individuals and social groups" (p. 16)

Program, Organisation, Source	Situation or context What were the needs? Why were people using digital stories?	Outputs What did people produce or do?	Reported outcomes Short term Individual and micro (interpersonal)	Reported outcomes Medium term Meso (community)	Reported outcomes Ultimate Macro (societal)
				• "A system of networked knowledge and a constellation of networked power which spoke with a global insight, coherence and authority that any one of the nodes would not have been unable [sic] to achieve on its own" • "The networked nature of a process like Participate … informs those involved that they are not acting alone, and that their actions benefit and enable others in a dynamic, interactive sequence of challenges, changes and reforms which can lead to the improved quality of life for many across a wide terrain, and not just in the immediate vicinity of one's own engagement and struggle" (p. 17)	• "Movement from fragmentation to collective knowing" (p. 16)

Program, Organisation, Source	Situation or context What were the needs? Why were people using digital stories?	Outputs What did people produce or do?	Reported outcomes Short term Individual and micro (interpersonal)	Reported outcomes Medium term Meso (community)	Reported outcomes Ultimate Macro (societal)
Mapping Our Voices for Equality (MOVE) King County, WA, USA (Benson, 2012)	• "increase community members' understanding of health disparities and inequities, mobilize members, and advocate for policy changes." • "The overall goal of this project is to evaluate the impact of MOVE's digital stories on forum attendees and to assess if any community actions and policy changes occurred as a result of the forums"	• Community forums involving local residents, school representatives, and policymakers • Digital stories by local residents • Research evaluation of impact of digital stories on participants in community forums	• "Forum attendees perceived MOVE's digital stories as authentic." • "The Digital Stories illustrated the root causes of certain health disparities" (p. 24) • The digital stories "illustrated ... the everyday impacts that policy decisions have on the lives of community members"	• "Many attendees felt the stories enriched their understanding of health disparities and related a fresh perspective on health topics not typically captured in media" • "Examples of policy changes include the restoration of operating hours slated to be cut from a community center, and planning to pilot new school lunch policies at a local Elementary school" • "Initiation of plans for a mobile grocer to locate in a neighborhood with limited healthy food access"	• "Examples of community actions include the mailing of 250+ postcards from local Latinos to Washington legislators in favor of tobacco quitline services"

outcomes such as more inclusive policymaking, effective democratic process, social justice, and so on.

Our reading of Table 6.1 is that medium-term, relatively localised listening outcomes are perhaps the more common ones to achieve. While we acknowledge the limitations of the analysis in terms of the limited availability of relevant policy-focused studies and the many unknown and "unknowable" outcomes of digital storytelling, it is notable that all studies reported significant limitations in the extent to which digital storytelling initiatives and activities could effect sustainable macro-level change. In some cases (see for example, Collin, 2008) storytelling participants were re-oppressed or further disenfranchised by their experience of engaging with decision makers. Collin's study of outcomes of digital participation for young people also found that existing inequities in terms of access to "voice" and influence were reproduced in the online policy participation setting. In others, storytellers and storytelling facilitators both reported the "glass ceiling" effect in that they felt they had achieved some positive intrinsic benefits such as a "feel good" atmosphere and local community building but had not achieved wider reach beyond their local community and networks (see Dreher, 2012).

Notably, it is the ultimate macro-level outcomes included in Table 6.1 that are often uncritically espoused in more utopian accounts of digital storytelling (e.g. promoting democracy, giving people a voice) without much attention to the contexts within which digital storytelling advocacy occurs, "how" these outcomes will be achieved, or the short- and medium-term outcomes that may be required to build towards ultimate macro-level outcomes. With exceptions, the reviewed literature describes that digital stories can be used in policy settings in anecdotal ways that do not allow for in-depth consideration of and response to the issues storytellers are raising. As Thea Shahrokh and Joanna Wheeler (2014) stated in regard to the Participate network's attempts to influence the post-2015 international development agenda, storytelling facilitators and participants often experience a risk that "Words and agendas generated through the [participatory] process [will] be co-opted and utilised to further existing agendas driving rather than transforming inequality and poverty" (p. 18). The existing literature we have surveyed here appears to support this fear that existing agendas will not be substantially transformed through processes associated with digital storytelling and advocacy. The literature reflects that while transformative outcomes may be achieved at a local level over relatively short time frames (see for example, Collin, 2008; Dreher, 2012), storytellers, advocates, and researchers can experience a glass ceiling effect when it comes to sustainably transforming institutional power and decision making via digital storytelling with marginalised people. This was particularly the case in policymaking in government institutions as opposed to non-government organisations which have been found to be more responsive and genuinely participatory (Collin, 2008). Further, Shahrokh and Wheeler found that systems and structures of decision making were sometimes inherently exclusive of "everyday" people's voices:

For many in the policymaking process, the idea of participation was understood as "consultation" or "listening to the poor". The gap between this and an understanding of participation as transformative of development was vast. This created a tension: we were trying to advance the understanding of participation and at the same time we were trying to gain acceptance of the importance of even rudimentary forms of participation ... [this produced] a tension around the adequate and authentic representation of highly marginalised groups within a system that is structured to exclude them ... the transformative potential of participatory knowledge is tied to its roots and the way in which it is grounded in the context that is [*sic*] was constructed in. In itself, this type of knowledge provides a complex challenge to the current development paradigm.

(Shahrokh & Wheeler, 2014, p. 19)

Agents within these decision-making systems and structures may request that stories, story-related content, and even storytellers be translated into a form that suits the dominant discourses and ways of seeing, being, and acting in elite policymaking and governance settings in order to be "listenable". This can occur with or without conscious recognition of the movements of power associated with these mediations.

Digital stories as one element of broader advocacy campaigns

While it is not frequently foregrounded in existing literature, our conversations with international digital storytelling practitioners, advocates, policymakers, and researchers revealed that digital stories are being used successfully as *just one part* of larger advocacy campaigns. Later in this chapter we consider the Ban Advocates initiative hosted by Handicap International as an example of how digital stories are being used as just one part of a broader strategic, international advocacy and media campaign to influence policymaking. Likewise, the Participate network on international development (see http://participate2015. org/) has, for example, been using digital stories as one strategy within a broader approach to having the voices of people living in poverty included in international decision making around international sustainable development goals. Other strategies employed by the Participate network include: participatory video; community radio; international participatory research projects; visiting fellowships; websites, blogs, and Twitter communications; written policy briefings; a documentary film; an exhibition in New York; written reports; Ground level panels and training; and communications and advocacy towards the UN Post-2015 High Level Panel of Eminent Persons (see Shahrokh & Wheeler, 2014).

In the context of the existing literature and interview findings outlined above we now turn to our two case studies for this chapter: the NDIS in Australia and the international Ban Advocates Initiative. We observe that the case studies both confirm and contradict the findings of existing studies presented in Table 6.1.

Case study: The National Disability Insurance Scheme (NDIS) Australia

The introduction of the Australian National Disability Insurance Scheme (NDIS) provides an interesting case study of how digital stories were gathered with a view to influencing policy in Australia. The case study explores life-story telling in the development of the NDIS in Australia. The following NDIS case study was developed through our joint analysis of publicly available documents and websites during 2012. Ethics approval was not required for this research.

A key component of NDIS policy development was the use of stories by various stakeholder groups, firstly to highlight the nature of the lived experiences of people with disabilities and their families and, secondly, to lobby for change. The notion of a national redesign of disability support arose from a widening concern that people with disability experienced vast unmet needs and experienced inequitable non-integrated services across state lines. A range of disability organisations and advocates hence launched a national movement to introduce an NDIS to reduce duplication and red tape between state and federal services and respond more effectively to the lived experiences and needs of all people with disabilities. A key component of this policy agenda was the use of stories by various stakeholder groups in their advocacy and lobbying efforts. Similar storytelling, albeit limited in scope, has been used in Australian disability policy processes for several years. The *Shut Out* report (National People with Disabilities and Carer Council, 2009) for example drew upon life story vignettes submitted to a previous Australian Senate inquiry.

We consider here the ways in which life narratives were treated as a resource for policymaking in the formulation of the NDIS. The NDIS case study points towards both the affordances of digital life stories and the challenges of listening to these accounts in the policymaking process. We focus in particular on two story collections established to influence the NDIS policy process. The first, *Your Story* – no longer available online – was instigated by the government agency and the second, *Every Australian Counts* (see http://www.everya ustraliancounts.com.au/), emerged from a broader coalition of interest groups (Butteriss, 2014; Thill, 2015).

The NDIS Your Story website

The NDIS *Your Story* website encouraged story submissions from a range of stakeholders including people with disability, family members, professionals, and paid carers. The "Your Story" guest book allowed registered users to submit their stories from mid-August 2012, though it is no longer available online. Participants were asked to comment on what they would expect from an NDIS within a limit of 250 words – a prescriptive and directive brief. The guest book invited video or photos but the site did not have an obvious mechanism for downloading or uploading them. The process had no pre-moderation of comments – stories could be put straight on – but within two hours they were moderated around the clock by administrators and filtered to identify high-risk language such as racist comments or ableist language. Administrators had authority to remove comments but much of the process was not clear and there were no clear ethical guidelines about participation. The site used a search tool but does not search content of stories for key words.

The Every Australian Counts website

Every Australian Counts was a people's campaign across the country, demanding the introduction of an NDIS, as recommended by the Productivity Commission. As such it was not government sponsored but rather relied on the contributions of service provider organisations, advocacy groups, and ordinary citizens. This campaign used a range of ICT technologies such as an interactive website, Facebook, Twitter, etc. There were two components to this collection. First, five stories were posted on the main site. These were carefully crafted and clearly selected for political purposes, reflecting "representative" lives of disabled people. These stories were in text format with a headshot photo of each person. The second repository on the site was an archive/blog including text, video, photos, blogs, and letters. The narrators here included people with disability and parents. It privileged text and some photos, with some videos, interspersed with video/text content about promoting the NDIS. This collection used tags, allowed for commentary, and included blogs from campaign coordinators, comments from celebrities, politicians, etc. Here the main focus was on the service system so that the lived experiences of people were mainly examined in relation to that system.

The visible movements of digital stories in the NDIS

Several dimensions of the story creation processes visible in the NDIS consultation are significant for listening in the context of policymaking. Clearly, both the *Your Story* and *Every Australian Counts* websites used public displays of collected digital stories to imply that their activities were centred around people's actual lived experiences. Collected digital stories were strongly portrayed as enacting a political, democratic, and inclusive movement of meanings between people with disabilities and a broader policy and decision-making audience. For example the website stated:

> People with disability, their families and carers must be at the centre of this reform. Your stories, experiences and aspirations will help reform disability care and support in Australia.

As a representation of a wider social movement for people with disabilities in Australia, the *Every Australian Counts* website featured five personal stories of people with disabilities and families prominently on its website. These stories were strongly "on message" in promoting the NDIS. For example, the five stories included a section on "what the NDIS would mean to me". Most of these stories elevated the importance of the NDIS beyond the personal to a broader "social good", as evident in the following excerpts from three of the stories:

> An NDIS is so important because it gives everybody a fair go and that's what being Australian is all about. I want to contribute to my community, to do that I need support in place. The NDIS will support me as an individual. It will give me a quality of life.
>
> (Claire)

> An NDIS is important because it can stop you having to fight for things. The biggest barrier for people with a disability is having to battle for every thing they need.
>
> (Peter)

> The most important thing is that with an NDIS Robert would be able to choose what works for him. The NDIS would mean that there would be a system in place that would have the funds to help people with disabilities.
>
> (Robert and Mary)

It is not clear how these five stories were selected or gathered apart from the fact that they appear to be professional-standard multimedia artefacts. Notably the *Every Australian Counts* website also encouraged people with disabilities to tell their story directly to politicians and policymakers and promoted the political power of collective voices. This invoked a mixture of both "static" voices that are encapsulated and represented via digital stories and more dynamic face-to-face and alternatively mediated (e.g. email) interactions with decision makers. For example a request to participants to write to their MP stated:

> Whether your story is brief or detailed when you put all of them together they form a picture of the huge numbers waiting for an NDIS, and what it's like to be in that holding pattern. And in putting stories to the numbers it makes the personal political.

The *Every Australian Counts* site also allowed more flexibility than the *Your Story* site in the length of stories that may be submitted or told. A more open process was also evident in the *Join the Conversation* news archive of this website. These postings included text, video, photos, blogs, letters, and media releases. There was opportunity for interactive dialogue and commentary and most postings had at least one comment or response. Many of these were made by people with disability or families, especially in response to government announcements regarding the NDIS.

What are the invisible movements of meaning in the NDIS?

What is less clear in both sites is what was done to and with the stories once they were submitted. This moment of mediation is a key and complex element of the adoption of digital stories in policy contexts. It is also unclear who was responsible for mediating the collected stories and the degree to which story-tellers may be re-engaged in decision-making and advocacy processes in the future. Lack of transparency in the policymaking process placed the reception of these digital stories in a "black box". The question of how a very large number of stories are collated and used is particularly interesting here. *Every Australian Counts* clearly saw the power of *multiple* stories influencing political processes and used these to further its campaign; however, the methods through which large numbers of stories might be mediated and listened to by policymakers were not described.

These two story-gathering activities raise some important questions about the processes involved in soliciting stories and their implications for listening. Significantly, several storytellers communicated their feelings about the limits of existing storytelling templates:

> 250 words is hardly enough to describe the difficulties we face as carers of someone with a mental illness.
>
> (Annie, 25 Sept)

> This is just the "tip of the iceberg" of my story.
>
> (Dreambear, 24 Sept)

> I am writing a book about this involvement with these beautiful people. … It seems that all the talk and stories are only heard by families with disabled children and then the stories dissolve away and go no further. I am attempting to bring to the public and governing bodies that these stories are real.
>
> (Dennis D, 27 Sept)

These accounts clearly emphasised that the templates for collecting narratives – and indeed the preconceptions by narrators of what makes a "listenable" story – shaped the range of narratives that could be listened to in very significant ways. While there was no directive to frame "your story" in a particular way, there was a very consistent pattern in the way these "stories" were told in both fora. For example, more than half of the contributors to "Your Story" chose in the opening sentences of their narrative to identify their impairment/s, often through a diagnostic label, or alternatively, describe their relationship (for instance, mother, partner, carer) to a person with a disability who is similarly identified through an impairment or diagnostic label.

We move next to discuss a case study of the use of digital storytelling in policymaking in which, thanks to detailed evaluation reports and interviews with advocacy organisations, it is possible to gain some insights into the way in which autobiographical narratives have shaped international policy. While the Ban Advocates example does not entirely open out the "black box" of policy, the fact that this is a long-standing campaign which has ultimately attained some of its policy objectives, enables us to have some "peep holes" into the process by which autobiographical narratives have been used by advocacy organisations and listened to by policymakers, this time at an intergovernmental level.

Case study: The Ban Advocates Project, Handicap International

The following case study was prepared using documentary and multimedia evidence available in the public sphere in addition to documents provided by Handicap International. It was also supplemented by in-depth interviews in 2016 and correspondence between 2012 and 2016 with Handicap International project staff responsible for the Ban Advocates initiative. Formal interviews were conducted under an ethics protocol approved via Griffith University.

Ban Advocates (BAs), associated with Handicap International, have been active in using digital life stories as part of advocating for international bans on the use of cluster munitions. The project includes advocates from Afghanistan, Albania, Croatia, Ethiopia, Iraq, Lao PDR, Lebanon, Serbia, Tajikistan, the USA, and Vietnam. Cluster munition and landmines victims include all persons directly impacted by cluster munitions as well as their affected families and communities. Advocates included people directly and indirectly affected by cluster munitions and landmines including people who had been directly injured and their family members. This case study traces the circulation and screening of the BAs' stories through social media and international diplomatic meetings and conferences, identifying the strategies behind the use of individual and collective narratives.

The BAs project is ultimately a success story of how networked advocacy and storytelling can support international-level change in the form of the adoption of the *Convention on Cluster Munitions* (henceforth "the Convention", see CMC, n.d.). The BAs' personal storytelling particularly influenced the inclusion of provisions for supporting victims of landmines and cluster munitions in the 2008 *Convention*. In the words of the Cluster Munition Coalition (CMC):

> The Convention on Cluster Munitions (CCM) is an international treaty that addresses the humanitarian consequences and unacceptable harm to civilians caused by cluster munitions, through a categorical prohibition and a framework for action. The Convention prohibits all use, production, transfer and stockpiling of cluster munitions. In addition, it establishes a framework for cooperation and assistance to ensure adequate care and rehabilitation to survivors and their communities, clearance of contaminated areas, risk reduction education and destruction of stockpiles.
>
> (CMC, n.d., n.p.)

The BAs project was formed after the 1997 *Mine Ban Treaty* (MBT; see United Nations, 1997) already existed. The BA project objective was hence to target cluster munitions in addition to landmines which were already covered under the MBT. Once the 2008 Convention was passed, the BAs project expanded to include victims of both landmines and cluster munitions. The BAs continued advocating for the universalisation and implementation of both the 1997 and 2008 treaties, in particular victim assistance obligations and international cooperation. We explore some of the mechanisms of this change below as well as some of the key characteristics of the BAs' work.

A long-term international campaign

The BAs project was part of the CMC (see http://www.stopclustermunitions.org/en-gb/home.aspx) formed to advocate for the adoption of a treaty against cluster munitions. The CMC:

> works through its members to change government policy and practice on cluster munitions – especially through promoting universal adherence to and full compliance with the 2008 Convention on Cluster Munitions – as well as to raise public awareness of the problem and the ban treaty through civil society campaigns and the media.
>
> (CMC, n.d., n.p.)

In 2011 the CMC campaign merged with the existing Nobel Peace Prize-awarded International Campaign to Ban Landmines (ICBL) to become the ICBL-CMC (see http://www.icblcmc.org/). The ICBL began in 1992 as a partnership between Handicap International, Human Rights Watch, Medico International, Physicians for Human Rights, Vietnam Veterans of America Foundation, and the Mines Advisory Group. It has since grown to include non-government organisations from over 100 countries and is ongoing in its efforts to support the human rights of landmine and cluster munitions survivors and their families (ICBL, n.d., n.p.).

Like many major social justice policy and legislative changes we have witnessed in Australia, the Convention has taken decades to bring into force. While the Convention was adopted in 2008 the ICBL-CMC and BAs' advocacy work is ongoing to ensure universal adherence to the principles set out in the Convention. This is perhaps one of the most important lessons to learn from the BAs project: major policy-level change does not often happen quickly or easily. Instead, it is often the result of decades of work by dedicated networks of advocates, champions, and policymakers who successfully influence diverse and multiple systems of decision making. Hence, we can immediately see that the "leap of faith" phenomenon often witnessed in digital storytelling literature and project reporting, that the simple act of telling stories will result in policy-level change, requires significant scrutiny.

Authenticity and voice in policymaking settings

In the previous chapters we have troubled the notion of promoting authenticity, agency, and control for storytellers while pursuing "applications" of their stories in institutional and community settings. Jeanne Battello, Handicap International former project officer for the BAs project, maintains that there is a strong link between storytelling and authenticity of voice for victims, even in complex advocacy that seeks to influence the highest levels of international governance:

> Stories can be, I think, used to influence both policy *making* [i.e. the creation of new policy] ... and when you want to change a policy that is existing and make it into something more specific or more accurate ... it's also a powerful tool, because it's authentic. What people are sharing is real, is the real world. It's their experience ... I think [with] the example of victims of landmines or cluster munitions, I think they are best placed to know what they need ... and they are best placed to tell us and to tell policy makers and to defend their rights.
>
> (Jeanne Battello, personal communication, 2016)

In many ways the BA project reaffirms the central tenets of classic digital storytelling with its emphasis on authenticity of voice. It is interesting that Handicap International has been able to promote these values of authenticity and representation while also achieving international influence via the MBT and CCM as part of the broader ICBL-CMC coalition. Battello also emphasises that when victims are engaged to talk about their lived experience of cluster munitions and landmines, they are the ones who will also be the primary beneficiaries of any change that results. This personal investment in the outcome of decisions that may flow from their activism significantly distinguishes them from other participants in negotiations and consultations. While many other participants in the CCM negotiations were there because of their technical knowledge or because of their formal authority as a country's diplomat or ambassador, the BAs were there to represent their own lives, families, and communities.

The BAs were part of an international network that came to powerfully represent the lived experiences of cluster munition victims both through their digital stories and through direct participation in international diplomacy processes around the 2008 Convention. This was verified by an independent evaluator of the Handicap International BAs project who found that:

> the Ban Advocates (BAs) were a vital factor contributing to the success of the Oslo Process. Their particular contribution, as part of the wider civil society campaign, was to help: Increase the legitimacy of the Oslo Process (along with affected countries); Strengthen the power of the humanitarian argument in favour of a ban; Influence diplomats understanding and

views of the issue, and in some cases contribute to a change in government policy; Strengthen the text of the convention, particularly on victim
assistance; Secure high profile media coverage for the Oslo Process; and
Motivate campaigners and diplomats.

(Mayne, 2009, p. 5)

Hence we can see that the BAs were involved in multiple dimensions of policymaking and related work during the lead-up to the Convention. This included
directly influencing the actual content of the Convention, especially on victim
assistance, and other activities surrounding its creation such as motivating
and inspiring other delegates and participating in media interviews. The BAs and
Handicap International have remained involved in subsequent international
activism to ensure that the Convention's signatories pursue its principles and
actions through domestic policy and law. They also continue to work for
broader adoption of the Convention by lobbying non-signatories.

Multimedia and multi-platform advocacy: digital stories as one part of a broader strategic approach

The BAs project can be defined in many ways through its multiplicity. It
resulted from collaboration with multiple non-government organisations
internationally through the ICBL-CMC, adopted multiple advocacy strategies
across multiple delivery platforms, and brought together multiple landmine
and cluster munitions victims to act as advocates and representatives for victims
in their own countries. In specific reference to digital stories, the BAs project
used a wide range of advocacy and storytelling activities across online and
offline settings. These included: creating digital documentaries and stories to
foster public awareness for the campaign and provide inspiration to other
victims; in-person storytelling tours in participating countries where digital
stories were circulated to promote events; direct participation in bilateral
meetings including the Oslo process which resulted in the Convention; written
communications to national government officials and diplomats which included
links to digital stories and documentaries; direct participation in smaller in-
person meetings with national government officials and diplomats in their
own countries; petitions; and media interviews and press releases which
included links to digital stories and documentaries.

Within this range of activities, Jeanne Battello observed that a key use of
the BAs' digital stories and documentaries was to develop public awareness
and mobilisation around banning and removing landmines and cluster munitions. This public awareness-raising and mobilisation was intended to put
pressure on decision makers to adopt and then sign the Convention and
undertake the actions it set out within their own countries. Decision makers
often heard BA members' stories repeatedly through diverse media sources
including face-to-face communication, media interviews, and so on. Hence,
we have an interesting example where the BA members' *digital* stories may

have never been directly "listened to" by decision makers themselves. Rather, the digital stories were used as part of a broader cross-platform online and offline campaign to influence the general public who would in turn place pressure on decision makers to act.

We found a similar use of digital stories to elicit public awareness and put pressure on governments in our conversation with Australian Media Officer for NGO ActionAid, Holly Miller. Holly's work often responds to women's needs in emergencies such as Cyclone Pam in Vanuatu and the typhoon in the Philippines. When we asked Holly about how she uses digital stories in her advocacy work, she explained:

> I think organisationally the incentive for doing any kind of media work and using people's stories to secure media coverage is to raise the profile of the organisation, but also then to put further pressure on government if we have got objectives at a particular point, and then also to attract attention to the work of the organisation ... and to therefore kind of increase our fundraising ... A lot of our media strategy, our communications, we're speaking to gain government attention and increase pressure on them to allocate resources to that thematic area.
>
> (Holly Miller, personal communication, 2016)

In a parallel story, participatory researcher Beth Cross of the University of West of Scotland collaborated with people with disabilities to create digital stories about the Scottish *Adult Support and Protection Act.* In Cross's words, the *Adult Support and Protection Act* (Scottish Government, 2007) deemed that local authorities "have a duty to investigate risk for adults who are deemed less able to safeguard their own well-being for any number of reasons ... we made these videos to take snapshots of the process of Adult Support and Protection from first concern that there might be a risk, through to how the person is left as the case closes" (Beth Cross, personal communication, 2016). The videos were then shared via training workshops and a partner NGO's website to be used as a resource for training disability workers. Within a year the video stories "were the highest hits that that organisation's whole site got" (Beth Cross, personal communication, 2016). Perhaps most interestingly for our purposes here, because of the success of the video stories via the website, the Scottish Government "basically adopted it [and] put those resources on the Scottish government website" (Beth Cross, personal communication, 2016). In Beth's words:

> So it went from, this is kind of radical, marginal research that the third sector has funded, to the Scottish government really embraced it. They had us come speak twice to ... their health and social care forums. So we were addressing the heads of all the major services and they were really pleased at the extent of the disabled researchers involved in it.
>
> *Naomi: So do you feel that you were influencing service delivery here or policy or both?*

Both ... One of the things that I think arose out of that is that they said each local authority has to have an independent advisory committee and the chair of that cannot be from within the social work department. It has to be an independent chair. So I ... felt that they [the video stories] were clearly instrumental in [leading to the Government] saying, we want to hear.

(Beth Cross, personal communication, 2016)

What seems to be emerging from our interviews with digital storytelling practitioners and researchers, then, is that a groundswell of public or service provider response to digital stories can lead to policymakers taking action in various ways – either directly or indirectly. These avenues of influencing policy are not well documented in the existing literature about digital storytelling.

The rise of social media with its potential for quickly distributing multimedia testimonies has no doubt enhanced the capacity of advocacy organisations to work in the ways described above. This notion of indirect political influence picks up on the theme of many-to-many forms of distribution evident in existing accounts of the political influence of digital storytelling, but sees this not simply as a democratising end in itself, but also as a step in a further political process. The movements of stories across social media, civil society, and various public arenas suggested in these accounts from Battello, Miller, and Cross constitute a more complex understanding of the effectiveness and power of digital stories, however, than simple empathetic connection between distant people.

Networked advocacy: beyond one voice

In considering the success of the BAs project we also need to overtly recognise the networked advocacy approach that was used. In their 2013 reflections on *Good Practice and Lessons Learned in Influencing Policy*, Handicap International emphasise the multiplicity of organisations and agents who contributed to the positive outcomes achieved in Oslo through the 2008 Convention:

The achievement of a diplomatic agreement and policy on the ban of cluster munitions was not due to an isolated campaign or event. It was the result of "strategic advocacy" and a tactical alliance of actors, the Cluster Munition Coalition (CMC) in particular, comprised of a global network of 350 civil society organisations working across 90 different countries.

(Handicap International, 2013, p. 10)

Jeanne Battello also emphasised that networked advocacy such as the ICBL-CMC is vital in moving beyond the "one story" approach to influencing policy. The "one story" approach is one where a single, often high-profile, storyteller comes to be seen as an archetypical case and thus inappropriately captures the attention of policy and decision makers at the expense of listening to other diverse storytellers and experiences. The BAs project has put a lot of time into developing what they call "representative" storytelling by the BAs themselves, i.e. that the individual Advocates from each participating country could act as representatives of their affected communities and also have opportunities to give back to those communities through the project:

> I think when you used story to do policy making, it needs to be some-how – the person that is calling on for policy change, needs not to be just individual. It needs to be representative of people that are behind the community or have a legitimate voice, otherwise I think the link, that cannot be made and it cannot really influence policy itself ... it's just one person trying to influence something.
>
> (Jeanne Battello, personal communication, 2016)

This networked advocacy and storytelling approach has interesting parallels to the calls for "big data" approaches to storytelling, research, and policymaking we have discussed previously (see Matthews & Sunderland, 2013). In effect, large coalitions of NGOs are using collections of digital stories and networks of storytellers to impress upon decision makers the breadth and significance of social and environmental issues being faced. While these story collections may or may not include enough stories to be quantifiably "generalisable" to an entire population, the focus on *representation* across diverse countries has been a significant element of the BAs' and broader CMC's success. The representative approach to storytelling upheld in the BAs project hence appears to assuage a common critique regarding the "danger of a single story" in shaping policy or other decision making (see for example, Adichie, 2009, n.p.).

"Changing the rules of the game"

With the backdrop of current literature on digital stories and policymaking provided earlier in this chapter, it is satisfying to find that diplomats involved in the Oslo process experienced an interruption to their normal ways of working due to the involvement of the BAs. According to one participant involved in the process:

> The BAs put them [the diplomats] in a dilemma – they either looked really bad or agreed with the BAs. The BAs simplified things down to the bare bones and changed the "rules of the game" for the diplomats.
>
> (participant quote, in Mayne, 2009, p. 9)

Within UN-based decision making there is an overt discourse on "expert" involvement that relates to the use and discourses of "expert panels" and so on. Experts are typically involved based on "technical" expertise rather than direct lived experience. As Shahrokh and Wheeler (2014) observe:

The consideration of "whose knowledge counts" in decision-making is significantly biased towards a centrally driven UN-level process, which entails emphasis on certain forms of "technical and expert" knowledge, and elite powerholders who are far removed from the realities of living in poverty.

(p. 8)

In our conversations with Jeanne Battello, she emphasised that the BAs' involvement in the broader international conversation around cluster munitions introduced a "different form of expertise" that was authentic and based on lived experience. Digital media artefacts used in the campaign also, according to Battello, actively reimaged the BAs from victims to champions and activists who took on esteemed leadership roles in their own countries, which shows perhaps unexpected positive mediations that occurred through the project.

Diplomats involved in the Oslo discussions leading to the Convention indicated respect for the BAs' specific knowledge and experience which indicates that they were seen as "experts" alongside others involved in the process:

> The BAs were experts in the human effects of CMs [cluster munitions] ... they brought specific experience which helped in the elaboration of the Victim Assistance clause ... I learnt a lot from them as they could tell me how things work on the ground and they raised several things I hadn't thought of.
>
> (diplomat's quote, in Mayne, 2009, p. 15)

Other international advocacy networks have similarly remarked on the inclusion of lived experience as a different form of expertise in UN-level negotiations and decision making. As Bivens articulates in relation to the Participate network and advocacy around post-2015 development goals, "Poor and excluded people also possess knowledge; knowledge rich with an understanding of their situations that policymakers and other advocates often fail to connect with" (Bivens, 2013, in Shahrokh & Wheeler, 2014, p. 17). The opening up of whose and which knowledge was valued in decision making in the Oslo process is arguably a real example of anti-oppressive and social justice outcomes that are possible from digital storytelling and related advocacy work. As we explore below, though, the elite expert decision makers involved in the process did not uniformly respond openly to the BAs' stories, which again moderates the extent to which we can claim any magical social justice-making process or outcome associated with digital storytelling in and of itself.

The limits and uses of empathy and emotion

The independent evaluator of the BAs project remarked on the limits of empathy in getting diplomats involved in the Oslo process to receive and act upon the BAs' experiences and recommendations:

experience from this and other campaigns suggests that emotional engagement is unlikely to be sufficient on its own if there are strong opponents, if states are heavily influenced by powerful vested interests, if the issue is highly contentious, and/or if there is lack of public support. In such cases high profile media coverage, public mobilisation, or other forms of pressure will also be necessary to achieve change.

(Mayne, 2009, p. 14)

Jeanne Battello also reported that project members were highly cognisant of the limits of empathy and emotion in the decision making process. Yet, while workers were aware of the limits of empathy and emotion, Battello reported:

While I was not at the negotiations, my colleagues' reports of the event indicate the BA's involvement was really striking … They [diplomats] were focused on technical aspects [and then] all of a sudden heard a human voice with an authentic story to tell … a true voice to … explain to them that it was going well beyond simply regulating arms … This … shows the emotion it can create and the impact it can create when you speak person to person.

(Jeanne Battello, personal communication, 2016)

Two diplomats involved in the Oslo negotiations confirmed Battello's impression of the impact that the BAs' stories had on them and the broader negotiations:

The Ban Advocates personified the impact and consequences of using these weapons. When you are a diplomat or a military expert discussing the technical details of different weapons, this is very different from seeing the human consequences … The BAs got us away from victims as numbers which do not mean much on a human level. It was much more powerful that the BAs were present in the form of living people.

(diplomat quote, in Mayne, 2009, p. 6)

While the above quotations are positive in reinforcing the value of BAs' participation and stories, a variable response from diplomats was known and understood by the BAs. Battello also observed that some diplomats involved in meetings following the adoption of the Convention were immediately responsive to the BAs and sought them out personally after formal meetings while others did not seem to react in a strongly personal way to the BAs' stories.

While the BAs' independent evaluator and Handicap International staff recognised the limits of empathy and emotion working on some diplomats involved in the Oslo process decision making, Battello also remarked on the power of emotional and empathetic responses to the BAs' digital stories and documentaries in speaking to other landmine and cluster munitions victims and members of their communities:

It was also giving people the opportunity to share with the broader community and to their peers and tell them, okay, I was like this at the beginning and now I became like that and this is the evolution that I had to make and it was difficult. Sometimes it has been a struggle, but it showed also other people that it was possible and something was possible there. I think it was inspiring. Like, the empathy it created from people that were not affected was strong. But for people that were affected, it was also displaying a role model for those external people that were evolving around the Ban Advocates themselves.

(Jeanne Battello, personal communication, 2016)

This more proximal social impact of the stories within the storytellers' own community affirms some of the literature reviewed in Table 6.1 in terms of the power of digital stories to evoke a localised "feel good" and community network-building response.

The favouring of "proactive" stories

When we talked with Australian former state government policy advisor, executive, academic, writer, and long-time disability activist Dr Donna McDonald about her use of stories in policymaking we asked her what kinds of stories worked best in policymaking in her experience. Without hesitation Donna replied: "The stories that work best are the stories that have a happy ending." With sentiments similar to the primary health care practitioners we spoke to in Chapter four, Donna explained:

No one likes to feel guilty or unhappy but no one wants – and this in fact was I think, now I'm thinking it through, was the dilemma of the disability movement for all those years – the whole guilt trip. You know, "we're isolated and lonely and alienated and we don't have anything and you make us feel terrible and you're the oppressors." That lets the oppressor [think] "well, okay, well we'll just oppress away" but we don't know what to do, and you're not giving us a way out here ... That's something any health minister likes to hear, a good way forward. So the best stories help you solve a problem or they reframe an old issue.

(Donna McDonald, personal communication, 2016)

It was quite striking then to also read the BAs project Independent Evaluator's conclusion that: "The moral force of affected individuals is increased when they come across as people who are positive and proactive, and want to help others, rather than just being victims to be pitied" (Mayne, 2009, p. 15). As indicated above, the Handicap International project officers had worked with the BAs to create a digital documentary where the BAs were actively positioned as champions and activists rather than "victims". This finding speaks to our earlier discussion of "listenable" stories in Chapter four where story facilitators actively screened and selected stories that weren't "ranty" or negative with hospital administration boards and staff. While this selectivity around choosing positive and "listenable" stories tweaks our own sense of discomfort and sensitivity about reproducing oppression and dominance through forum control, it is a reality and a key tension of contemporary listening environments that appears across a number of case studies and conversations presented in this book. We now turn to theorising the significance of these case studies.

Theorising listening

Voice, agency, and mediation in policymaking settings

As articulated in Chapter one, the bulk of existing work in digital storytelling emphasises giving or having a "voice" rather than listening to those voices. Proponents of digital storytelling often frame storytelling as being both beneficial and liberating for storytellers in areas such as political participation, self-expression, and skill development (Burgess, 2006; Hartley, McWilliam, Burgess, & Banks, 2008; Hull & Nelson, 2005; Rossiter & Garcia, 2010). But what happens to the notions of storyteller voice and agency when stories and potentially storytellers themselves enter into policymaking contexts as was the case in the BAs and NDIS case studies above?

Across all contexts of storytelling and listening we have encountered in this book there is a strong focus on maintaining "authenticity" of voice and seeing storytellers as "whole persons". Storytelling facilitators and researchers often extend this commitment to authenticity to attempting to keep personal stories "intact" by trying to respond to the story as a whole rather than deconstructing and mining stories for perceived relevant content. Surprisingly, this desire to keep stories intact is often the case even when dealing with very large numbers of stories. For instance, one of the few articles on digital storytelling to be based on a survey of a large number (200+) of digital stories nonetheless returns to a case study approach for its fine-grained account of the relationship between modes of communication (Hull & Nelson, 2005; see also Hartley et al., 2008). Similarly, large-scale social research projects that have sought to locate life narratives in terms of broader political and social history often present their findings in the form of case studies (see for example, Goodley, Lawthom, Clough, & Moore, 2004). In the case of the NDIS, specific organisations collected very large numbers of stories but the "black box" effect of what happened to those stories once they were collected has precluded us from being able to see how large numbers of stories were analysed and interpreted in the NDIS policymaking processes.

Some digital storytelling researchers and facilitators have also been critical of policymakers' and others' – such as journalists' – perceived tendency to summarise or mine stories and not engage with them as a whole. Lénárt-Cheng and Walker (2011), for instance, comment critically on one digital story hosting organisation's attempts to make the narratives in one image-based storytelling site more accessible to elites:

> On its web site, for example, Panos offers searchable summaries of individual testimonies. These shortened versions are supposed to be more accessible and useful to policymakers and journalists, who otherwise would never have the time to read the stories in their original length. But what is lost in these abridged versions is precisely the intimate voice of the single individual.
>
> (Lénárt-Cheng & Walker, 2011, p. 151)

Yet not all listening mediations surrounding policymaking will be inherently reductive or opaque. While it may be the case that some negative or limiting mediations of the BAs' stories were not visible to us, the BAs project appears to be one example where the authenticity of voice and integrity of story were not sacrificed by these mediating processes of "fitting in" to an existing institutional listening environment, i.e. the international Convention negotiation process.

Likewise, some researchers and activists have observed that individual storytellers can enhance their own political agency through being part of storytelling and listening activities. Rossiter and Garcia (2010), for instance, proclaim: "we believe that the long-term impact of digital storytelling is inextricably tied to individuals' access to thousands – indeed, millions – of viewers/listeners through the Internet" (p. 47). Implicit in Rossiter and Garcia's statement is an argument that large-scale shifts in public opinion can be enabled by one-to-many contact via the Internet. While we did not see evidence of such developments in individual agency via our two case studies, we did see examples in the BAs project and in Holly Miller and Beth Cross's work where public opinion was used – deliberately or inadvertently – as a lever to influence policymaking (personal communication). Jeanne Battello also noted that the individual BAs sometimes took on "celebrity" roles in their home countries and became the "go to" person for certain policy issues and discussions with their home government representatives, hence significantly enhancing their individual presence and, potentially, agency in that context. Furthermore, the continuing presence of the NDIS and BAs' stories in social media settings creates the possibility of relatively unknown or unknowable ongoing one-to-many dissemination and influence in the ways that Rossiter and Garcia (2010, p. 47) describe above.

Disrupting the status quo?

As we have prepared this book, we have realised more and more that digital storytelling proponents need to get real in questioning whether and how digital storytelling and listening are disrupting the existing status quo of privilege and oppression that leads to certain voices being elite and others marginalised. If this disruption to the existing dynamics of privilege and marginalisation is occurring, how is it occurring and what are its effects for people who experience oppression? We also have to get real about the possibility that attempts at enhancing participation may incur localised individual- or interpersonal-level change but may also actively reinforce the existing status quo at other meso and macro levels of activity. In her exploration of the policymaking impact of the Center for Digital Storytelling's Silence Speaks project in Africa, for example, Polk (2010) challenges digital storytelling proponents to consider how "emancipatory" and "authentic" digital storytelling can be if it adopts a Westernised cultural model of storytelling, such as the Center for Digital Storytelling (CDS) classical digital storytelling model. Polk further challenges us to critically evaluate how cultural differences are being addressed and upheld in storytelling projects and related listenings. Likewise, changes at the macro level, such as the international Convention in the BAs case, may or may not "trickle down" to influence domestic policy or the daily lived experiences for storytellers and their allies.

The questions outlined above are similar to issues we canvassed in Chapter four regarding the way listening intermediaries often feel the need to be strategic in selecting stories that are actionable and "palatable" for decision makers. Listening intermediaries may select stories that fit with the existing agenda of public board meetings, for instance, or which are framed in ways that avoid them being seen as "too ranty". However, we also saw in Pip Hardy's account of the reception by organisational listeners of Vanessa Lett's story "Thank you very much", the ways that even the most non-confrontational narratives can be read as a threat (personal communication). As we have indicated in Chapter four, the pressure to adapt or select the "right" stories that practitioners and policymakers are most likely to listen and respond to makes for a tense, complex, and problematic process given the social justice aims of digital storytelling generally. Silence Speaks has long-standing strategies for navigating these tensions. One strategy to navigate these tensions is not so much by adapting or selecting stories as framing them. Amy Hill spoke to us about the importance of developing the right collateral material that shows those audiences "What is it that you actually want me to do, what's the takeaway, what's the actionable item". Silence Speaks often draws on storytellers themselves to introduce and frame recorded stories as they are being presented to elite listeners. In other contexts, however, these frictions between the promise of an "unmediated" and "authentic" voice for storytellers and the realities of the way stories are funnelled into the existing ways of working and preferences of elite decision makers and professionals continue to be an often unacknowledged presence.

Other realities are also at play when we consider whether digital storytelling can lead to disruptions in the status quo. Participation in health policy often requires community representatives to take on practices that may be unfamiliar or inconvenient to them – for example, reading the formal minutes of meetings or policy documents. The intersections and influence of culturally and politically dominant and privileged habits of mind and activity – and the need for policymakers to allow themselves to be "put out" of their potentially normal and accepted ways of working – were particularly evident when we talked to Dr Donna McDonald. Donna's experiences in using storytelling in policymaking *as a policymaker* were simultaneously profound, disturbing, and affirming. Here we share an excerpt of one of the many stories Donna shared with us about her work in a state government department in Australia:

> My senior colleague [name] and I decided how about we – once we've got all the evidence and the advice in from all the government departments – how about we write up the cultural policy strategy, so we've had to do the strategy and the policy at the same time. How about we embed it with little micro narratives. It was warmly received by many government ministers and warmly received by the arts sector and they were intrigued that we tried to weave a narrative and use little mini micro stories, particularly from the rural sector. But [name of senior executive in department] pulled it the day before it went to Cabinet.
> Naomi: Pulled the whole document?
> Donna: Pulled the whole document. Later on she explained to me that she didn't really understand the approach of this narrative and she thought it was a bit "girly". She admitted she didn't have the confidence to sell it to her own Minister [name]. I still believe [minister's name] would have bought it. I still believe he would have carried it into Cabinet.
> Naomi: So we're dealing with privileged ways of knowing and representing.
> Donna: Privileged ways of knowing, privileged ways of representing, and also having the courage, or the lack thereof, to break through that privilege by people who should know better.
> (personal communication with Donna McDonald, 2016)

The inclusion of the pejorative "girly" stands out in Donna's story as affirmation that dominant ways of seeing, being, and working were at work, or perceived to be at work, in this policymaking setting to the point that her female senior executive refused to take the draft cultural policy to the state government's cabinet of all ministers for consideration and approval.

Yet we do not want to assume that marginalised storytellers are incapable of, or unused to, managing the dynamics of their interactions with elite decision makers. In many cases managing and responding to privileged and dominant ways of being, seeing, and doing is something that marginalised people do every day. As Goggin (2009) points out, many Deaf people and people with disabilities are expert at switching communication modalities in an attempt to elicit a more attentive listener. Other, more privileged, listeners are often less accustomed to the requirement to deploy a range of different strategies when listening. In the related context of intercultural communication, Hawkins and Downing suggest that competence in such contexts involves, "flexibility and learned ability to creatively tolerate ambiguity" (cited in O'Donnell, Lloyd, & Dreher, 2009, p. 425). It's interesting to note in this context that it is "open" stories – ones that contain ambiguities and unresolved dilemmas – that educators and "listening brokers" viewed as often most powerful for service improvement. Such stories may be more "palatable" than more confrontational accounts, but they also require the listeners to think through how they would respond to the professional dilemma or difficulty being presented, to think through and possibly shift their position. The often static nature of digital storytelling collections – the inability of these narratives to shift terrain in response to the favoured modes of communication of policymakers and other elite listeners – places the onus on privileged listeners to make such moves. Tanja Dreher (2009) formulated one form of listening which may be relevant to policy listenings to digital storytelling as "eavesdropping with permission" – a form of listening by privileged people who are used to dominating the conversation (p. 1).

Institutionalised listening

The familiarity and similarity of many of the stories produced for the NDIS "Your Story" guest book evoke Liz Stanley's (2002) account of life story telling as inextricably connected to genres of "official" life story telling such as clinical interviews. As Lorna Hallahan (2009) has pointed out, further, people with disability are often expected to tell and retell traumatic stories, stories of the worst things that have happened to them, in order to have maximal political effectivity. Applying for accommodation from welfare or educational systems often requires narrating one's areas of difficulty or incapacity, and one's most difficult moments. Particular stories are "coaxed" here by the requirements of particular listeners – or even by the expectation of particular kinds of listening on the part of listening storytellers alert to particular genres of story and types of narrative.

In the case of the BAs, Jeanne Battello commented that digital stories and other print communications were used strategically to inform decision makers and journalists prior to their face-to-face encounters with the BA representatives themselves. This was used as a mechanism for managing the strain on the storytellers in retelling potentially traumatic stories over and over again. Recruiting and supporting multiple storytellers – rather than just a single storyteller – was another technique that the BAs project officers used to manage storyteller fatigue and potential re-traumatisation.

The patterns to the stories told through the NDIS and BAs projects emphasise that the story hosts and caretakers, those who manage the medium through which stories are shared – the pathways of mediation between storytellers and their potential audiences – are significant players in an "ecosystem" of mediation and listening around personal experience. In the case of the NDIS guest book, while the requirement for a brief written text of the guest book imposed a form on these narratives, there was very little in the "brief" to write your story that might have led storytellers to so frequently turn to the form of the clinical narrative of impairment. Stories were not prompted or edited to go down this path, and yet very many of them did.

These case studies have potentially profound implications for how we conceptualise listening in relation to social change. We cannot simply conceptualise the "funnelling" process by which elite listeners narrow and channel stories as something that happens through the intervention of editors and other media professionals, gatekeepers and brief-writers, those listening brokers who select and foreground particular stories for attention. In framing their narratives, storytellers are already marshalling the narrative resources with which they are familiar – biomedical accounts of disability for instance, or the genre of the clinical case study – to offer a story for the kinds of listeners they anticipate will encounter their tale. Modes of listening, as well as genres of story, that are comfortable and familiar to elite listeners, "pre-populate" personal storytelling processes built into the policymaking process. This process, beautifully analysed in Anna Poletti's (2011) account of digital storytelling, and acknowledged by many of the digital storytelling practitioners we spoke to, runs counter to more utopian understandings of how digital storytelling might work to shift relations of power.

At the same time, the NDIS guest book offers a more hopeful perspective on the ways in which the invisible influence of anticipated listeners and their favoured modes of communication might be mitigated. Several self-identified Deaf contributors posted stories to the guest book which conformed with none of the characteristic features of the clinical narrative – no diagnostic labels or date of onset, no medical languages or treatments. The powerful frame offered by a vision of cultural Deafness – Deafhood as a unique way of experiencing the world to be celebrated not regretted, sign language as a community language, with associated requirements for community media, appropriate interpreters, and so forth – appeared to present an alternative narrative resource enabling these participants to tell their stories in ways that broke the unspoken rules of how to tell your NDIS story. These storytellers demanded alternative modes of listening to the biomedical problem-solving modality described by the patient experience managers we spoke to in Wales, as we discussed in Chapter four. The NDIS guest book example indicates that using digital stories to shape policymaking for social justice ends requires both a "hands off" approach to allow stories to be "freely" offered and allowance for diverse modes of storytelling. Moving beyond already-familiar genres and types of story may require explicitly declaring an openness to listening to different communication modes – Australian sign language video as well as written English for instance – and to different genres of stories as well. For instance, Lorna Hallahan (2009) has called for policymakers to hear stories of the "disabled everyday" rather than requiring stories of difficulty and trauma. Susan Bickford (1996) views this kind of ongoing openness as one of the key dimensions to political listening. It is challenging to reflect on the alternative modes of listening such stories might require. Equally challenging is imagining how an openness to a greater diversity of kinds of narrative might be clearly conveyed to potential storytellers.

At a broader level, we recognise the complexity of the task of promoting social change for social justice. In particular, we recognise that shifting centuries of privileged decision making and elitism in favour of anti-oppressive practice at any level of policymaking will not come easily. At a mundane practical level, policymaking timelines and time frames often do not match with the extended time frames required to engage in "authentic" and self-determined digital storytelling programs and projects (see for example, Shahrokh & Wheeler, 2014, p. 19). Likewise, systematic and complex evaluation of policy outcomes can be hindered by limited digital storytelling project budgets and time frames. There is also much complexity and heterogeneity to policymaking and advocacy practices and contexts which means it can be logistically difficult for digital storytelling participants, advocates, and researchers to effectively monitor and evaluate the extent to which a particular storytelling project or advocacy initiative has shaped policy outcomes.

These case studies suggest, though, that we need to think of the mediation of stories, and the role of listeners, as a negotiation between teller and listeners, a negotiation process, needless to say, in which elite listeners hold many – but not all – of the cards. Storytellers and their allies are often well equipped to manage and resist the systems of power and privilege that shape their daily existence. This acknowledgement makes the effective use of personal storytelling to rupture and reshape policymaking processes much more difficult, but also infinitely more hopeful.

Take-aways for practitioners

- While we are cautious not to overstate the impact of digital stories in policy, digital storytellers and their allies are influencing policymaking in direct and indirect ways, from the individual and interpersonal local level through to the macro level of international policy.
- While the bulk of academic literature reports stronger immediate listening outcomes at the interpersonal and community levels there are examples of digital storytelling and parallel processes being used successfully at the international policymaking level.
- Advocates and self-advocates often use digital storytelling as just one technique in a broader advocacy strategy. Advocates and self-advocates are also often working as part of broader networks of representative storytellers and their allies.
- Storytellers and their allies are often well equipped to manage and resist the systems of power and privilege that shape their daily existence and dominate many policymaking settings.
- Familiar and limited ways of telling personal stories can shape the way storytellers choose to frame the narratives they produce in policymaking forums. In seeking out stories, advocacy organisations and policymakers

need to explicitly indicate the openness of listeners to a diversity of modes of communication and types of story to help prompt a wider and more representative range of narratives.

- Simply inviting storytellers to tell "their story" will not necessarily produce an "authentic" or diverse collection of narratives, since storytellers often anticipate the kinds of listeners they may have and attempt to produce the sorts of stories that may be "listenable" to decision makers.
- Even with high levels of organisation and strategy, it takes many years and often decades to elicit policy-level change. Social change for health and well-being is a long-term and complex prospect but we can take hope from some current activities.
- Influencing policymaking is a complex task. There is a lot we still do not know about how digital stories are used in policymaking. This is because policymaking itself is a complex and often opaque process.
- It is possible that digital storytelling projects can elicit social change and social justice at one level – e.g. macro international policy – without achieving significant change at other levels in the health promotion continuum: in interpersonal relationships, service delivery, or domestic policy and law, and vice versa. Movements toward social change and social justice hence require networked attention across the health promotion continuum – i.e. across individual, interpersonal, meso, and macro levels – to ensure systemic and sustainable change in the social determinants of health.
- There are tensions in making stories "listenable" to by policymakers and retaining a focus on emancipation and authentic voice. These are not mutually exclusive categories, though, as evidenced in the Ban Advocates case study.
- Digital stories and other story media can assist in supporting storytellers and prevent burnout and re-traumatisation through having to repeatedly tell one's story to new listeners in policymaking and other settings.

Conclusion

This chapter traces the connection linking contemporary understandings of listening and storytelling to policymaking. Storytelling has become an important and much-publicised part of public consultation and participation in the policy process. What the advocacy projects and organisations examined in this chapter ultimately tell us is that digital storytelling's effect on policy-making needs to be seen, assessed, and planned in context. At this point in time, non-government advocacy organisations seem to be the most well-equipped organisations for influencing policy that we have spoken to. This conclusion is supported in the existing literature which indicates that participants feel more "intact" after engaging with non-government organisations as opposed to government organisations. We believe this is primarily because of NGOs' knowledge and embeddedness within policymaking circles and their "realistic" understandings of "the way things work" within those circles. Advocacy organisations are very strategic and deliberate in the ways they use digital stories and other media and content to achieve their aims. The advocacy organisations we spoke to also generally position policy-level change as their primary goal whereas other organisations that facilitate and share digital stories such as universities, broadcasters, or galleries may have other values and goals at the centre of their practice such as artistic expression, local community development, skills development, and so on.

References

Adichie, C. (2009). *The Danger of a Single Story.* TEDx talk. Retrieved from https://www.ted.com/talks/chimamanda_adichie_the_danger_of_a_single_story?language=en

Benson, S. (2012). *Exploring Digital Storytelling Applications in the Community: Implementation and Impact of Four Community Forums in King County, WA.* Retrieved from https://digital.lib.washington.edu/researchworks/handle/1773/20650

Bickford, S. (1996). *The Dissonance of Democracy: Listening, Conflict and Citizenship.* Ithaca, NY: Cornell University Press.

Burgess, J. (2006). Hearing ordinary voices: Cultural studies, vernacular creativity and digital storytelling. *Continuum: Journal of Media & Cultural Studies, 20*(2), 201–214.

Butteriss, C. (2014). Gathering rich personal stories online to inform the Australian National Disability Insurance Scheme. *Bang the Table: All about Engagement,* January 7. Retrieved from http://www.bangthetable.com/gathering-rich-personal-stories-online/

Cluster Munition Coalition (CMC) (n.d.). *Cluster Munition Coalition* [website]. Retrieved from http://www.stopclustermunitions.org/en-gb/the-treaty.aspx

Collin, P. (2008). The internet, youth participation policies, and the development of young people's political identities in Australia. *Journal of Youth Studies, 11*(5), 527–542.

Dreher, T. (2009). Eavesdropping with permission: The politics of listening for safer speaking spaces. *Borderlands E-Journal, 8*(1), 1–21. Retrieved from http://www.borderlands.net.au/vol8no1_2009/dreher_eavesdropping.pdf

Dreher, T. (2012). A partial promise of voice: Digital storytelling and the limits of listening. *Media International Australia, 142*(1), 157–166.

Flitcroft, K., Gillespie, J., Salkeld, G., Carter, S., & Trevena, L. (2011). Getting evidence into policy: The need for deliberative strategies? *Social Science & Medicine, 72*(7), 1039–1046.

Funkenstein, A. (1993). The incomprehensible catastrophe: Memory and narrative. In R. Josselson & A. Lieblich (Eds.), *The Narrative Study of Lives* (pp. 21–29). Newbury Park, CA: Sage.

Goggin, G. (2009). Disability and the ethics of listening. *Continuum: Journal of Media & Cultural Studies, 23*(4), 489–502.

Goodley, D., Lawthom, R., Clough, P., & Moore, M. (2004). *Researching Life Stories: Method, Theory and Analyses in a Biographical Age.* London: Routledge Falmer.

Hallahan, L. (2009, September 28–30). Public Testimony: Empowerment or humiliation? Paper presented at The Story of the Story: Life Writing, Ethics and Therapy Conference, Flinders University, Adelaide.

Handicap International (2013). *Advocacy with Victims: Good Practice and Lessons Learned in Influencing Policy* [report]. Retrieved from http://www.handicap-interna tional.org/wp-content/uploads/2016/09/DOC19_ENG.pdf

Hartley, J., McWilliam, K., Burgess, J. E., & Banks, J. A. (2008). The uses of multimedia: Three digital literacy case studies. *Media International Australia Incorporating Culture and Policy: Quarterly Journal of Media Research and Resources, 128*, 59–72.

Hernandez, M. (2000). Using logic models and program theory. *Education & Treatment of Children, 23*(1), 24–40.

Hull, G. A., & Nelson, M. E. (2005). Locating the semiotic power of multimodality. *Written Communication, 22*(2), 224–260. doi: 10.1177/0741088304274170

International Campaign to Ban Landmines (ICBL) (n.d.). *International Campaign to Ban Landmines* [website]. Retrieved from http://www.icbl.org/en-gb/home.aspx

Jones, M., & Einsiedel, E. (2011). Institutional policy learning and public consultation: The Canadian xenotransplantation experience. *Social Science & Medicine, 73*(5), 655–662.

Lénárt-Cheng, H., & Walker, D. (2011). Recent trends in using life stories for social and political activism. *Biography, 34*(1), 141–179.

Lundby, K. (Ed.) (2008). *Digital Storytelling, Mediatized Stories: Self-Representations in New Media*. New York: Peter Lang.

Matthews, N., & Sunderland, N. (2013). Digital life-story narratives as data for policy makers and practitioners: Thinking through methodologies for large-scale multimedia qualitative datasets. *Journal of Broadcasting & Electronic Media, 57*(1), 97–114.

Mayne, R. (2009). *External Evaluation of the Ban Advocates (BAs) Initiative: Summary of Findings and Lessons* [report]. Retrieved from http://issuu.com/handicap internationalbelgium/docs/banadvocates_ra2009

National People with Disabilities and Carer Council (2009). *SHUT OUT: The Experience of People with Disabilities and their Families in Australia*. Retrieved from http://www.fahcsia.gov.au/sa/disability/pubs/policy/community_consult/Pages/defa ult.aspx

Nutbeam, D., & Boxall, A. M. (2008). What influences the transfer of research into health policy and practice? Observations from England and Australia. *Public Health, 122*(8), 747–753.

O'Donnell, P., Lloyd, J., & Dreher, T. (2009). Listening, pathbuilding and continuations: A research agenda for the analysis of listening. *Continuum: Journal of Media & Cultural Studies, 23*(4), 423–439.

Poletti, A. (2011). Coaxing an intimate public: Life narrative in digital storytelling. *Continuum: Journal of Media & Cultural Studies, 25*(1), 73–83.

Polk, E. (2010). Folk media meets digital technology for sustainable social change: A case study of the Center for Digital Storytelling. *Global Media Journal, 10*(17), n.p.

Rossiter, M., & Garcia, P. A. (2010). Digital storytelling: A new player on the narrative field. *New Directions for Adult and Continuing Education, 126*, 37–48. doi: 10.1002/ace.370

Scottish Government (2007). *Adult Support and Protection (Scotland) Act 2007*. Retrieved from http://www.legislation.gov.uk/asp/2007/10/contents

Shahrokh, T., & Wheeler, J. (Eds.) (2014). *Knowledge from the Margins: An Anthology from a Global Network on Participatory Practice and Policy Influence*. Brighton: IDS.

Sillato, M. C. (2008). *Huellas: Memorias de Resistencia (Argentina 1974–1983)*. San Luis, Argentina: Nueva Editorial Universitaria.

Stanley, L. (2002). From 'self-made women' to 'women's made-selves': Audit selves, simulation and surveillance in the rise of the public woman. In T. Cosslett, C. Lury, & P. Summerfield (Eds.), *Feminism and Autobiography: Text, Theories, Methods* (pp. 40–60). London: Routledge.

Thill, C. (2015). Listening for policy change: How the voices of disabled people shaped Australia's National Disability Insurance Scheme. *Disability & Society, 30*(1), 15–28.

United Nations (1997). *Convention on the Prohibition of the Use, Stockpiling, Production and Transfer of Anti-Personnel Mines and on their Destruction.* Retrieved from http://legal.un.org/avl/ha/cpusptam/cpusptam.html

VeneKlasen, M. C., with Miller, V. (2007). *A New Weave of Power, People and Politics: The Action Guide for Advocacy and Citizen Participation.* Bourton on Dunsmore: Practical Action Publishing.

7 Hope, contradictions, and an interdisciplinary future

Digital storytellers and their allies set out to do extraordinary things – to amplify stifled voices, to enable the creation of new kinds of stories, to reshape hierarchies of expertise, and to tap into vital new insights on the world. The importance and difficulty of these tasks are not to be under-estimated. We admire and share these ambitions, and with them in mind, our aim in this book has been to map out and theorise the ways life experience narratives have been used to try to make social change happen in diverse health and social policy contexts. What we have uncovered gives us a renewed sense of hope, founded on the energy and persistence of storytellers and their allies around the world as they work towards social justice and health equity. This hope is sustained by what we have begun to see – the extent to which many decision makers and practitioners in health and social policy are already listening. Our exploration of the listening occasions in this book has been underpinned both by this sense of hope and by a belief that ambitions for equality and justice are best served by understanding the complexity of what it means to use digital stories, in health and social policy and elsewhere.

One way of framing digital storytelling in health and social policy is as a movement generated by outsiders to biomedicine, speaking back to elite voices and challenging their dominant framing of health and how it should best be achieved. This vision of digital storytelling as grounded in community activism, thriving outside corporate media and powerful state institutions, tells us important things about the origins of digital storytelling and the way it has played out in the first decades of the twenty-first century. But this account of community activism doesn't tell us everything we need to know. Our conversations with practitioners using digital storytelling to try to improve health and social policy – by changing professional education and shifting policy and practice – have suggested that a more complex story is at play.

Over the past thirty years, personal storytelling hasn't just become a staple on popular television and social media. It has also become a key element in public institutions', government, non-government, and professional organisa-tions' ways of working. With institutionalisation, though, come new dimen-sions to the unavoidable mediation of personal narratives: the filtering and reshaping of meanings to accord with institutional and organisational needs, strategies, and ways of working and seeing. This is not to say that organisations' and institutions' calls for stories are simply a public relations gesture, although at times they can be. Encouraging people to tell their personal stories has undoubtedly become, however, a key way in which organisations seek to demonstrate to both the public and government agencies their responsiveness and transparency. We saw this most clearly in Chapter four in our discussion of storytelling in the British National Health Service (NHS) and in Chapter six with the example of the consultation process for the Australian National Disability Insurance Scheme (NDIS).

Some professions, organisations, and institutions now have well-established strategies for listening to personal stories of health and well-being. The British Royal College of Nursing for example has been drawing out and reflecting on personal narratives in health care for decades. It has used these stories systematically and routinely as part of professional education and staff accreditation. Patient experience managers who collect and share patient stories to enhance service provision are now embedded in national health care systems such as the Welsh NHS. While community-based digital storytelling projects still take place around the globe, often these are commissioned, funded, or sponsored by councils, government departments, museums or libraries, universities, or other public institutions. Many of the stories we have shared in this book, then, have been stories of how multimedia personal storytelling might work inside, or in conjunction with, institutions and their existing hierarchies of power and expertise.

Not all health care professionals and policymakers systematically or thoughtfully listen to health consumers' stories. Even when listening happens, there is no guarantee that the ensuing action will result in health equity or social justice. Yet, we do not want to end this book with a call to those in positions of power to start listening to individuals' stories of health and health care. In many cases, they are already doing it. This listening may be compromised – occasional, distracted, cursory, or fragmented – but one way or another, it is happening in many places. The questions of how meaningful these occasions of listening are, and how effective they are at changing not just institutionalised practices but also the broader status quo, are questions we have begun to ask in this book. Increasingly, however, questions of how personal stories can be listened to in meaningful and impactful ways have come to be part of the way health services report on their activities and evaluate their successes.

There is a radical participatory impulse behind "specific" or "classic" digital storytelling and indeed many other practices of drawing on personal narrative for social justice ends. Proponents of anti-oppressive and emancipatory approaches to storytelling want to transform the flows and structures of knowledge and power: they do not want to simply give health service users the opportunity to be consulted occasionally at the discretion of elite decision makers. Yet even the staunchest radical activists and self-advocates would likely acknowledge that there are many ways to advocate for social change and that both a strategic and multifarious approach is required to prompt far-reaching and sustained shifts in power relationships. As critical social work scholars such as Christine Fejo-King and Linda Briskman (2009) and Jan Fook (2012) have emphasised, one size does not fit all when it comes to promoting social change and social justice across the health promotion continuum. The road to complex social change instead requires a matching complexity and plurality of approaches. As a result, we have used the phrase "digital storytelling" to capture many diverse and related practices across the health and social policy settings case studied in this book. Our aim has been to deliberatively draw together a wide and generative set of interdisciplinary and inter-professional digital storytelling and related practices for analysis and learning across boundaries.

One of our key moves in this book has been to view the contexts of listening as just as important as the stories themselves or the process – however liberatory or transformational – by which these stories are made. Our attention to the environments for listening introduced in Chapter two – including the meta-oratory roles of the listening curator, broker, caretaker, and host – allowed us to map out diverse ways that multimedia experiential stories are being circulated, framed, and used in health and social policy settings. In turn, this allowed us to consider what has and hasn't worked in promoting listening and response to personal digital storytelling. Our conclusions here can only be exploratory, not least because our observations and conversations suggest that the ways in which listening to digital stories plays out are embedded in particular places and spaces. As we have suggested elsewhere, the dissemination of digital stories has often been imagined as a process where one individual's life directly touches another's through the medium of a moving story (Matthews & Sunderland, 2013). In contrast, one of our key arguments here has been that overlapping ecosystems of meta-orators – not just facilitators, but caretakers, hosts, and brokers – need to be considered not as an unfortunate "impediment" to authentic and direct sharing of voice but, rather, as an inevitable and often critically important part of the way stories are moved to their listeners.

It is evident from our case studies that interpersonal, institutional, and geographical locatedness is a key dimension to understanding how listening might occur. This focus on the locations of listening is present in our emphasis on deep embodied and emplaced listening as a resource for meaning making. As we discussed in Chapter five, such deep embodied and emplaced listening is an everyday practice for people from many marginalised cultures that is now being taken up in the health and social policy system both as a therapeutic intervention and as a mode of organisational development and learning.

Throughout this book, we have learnt through conversations with policymakers, researchers, and storytelling facilitators, placing these perspectives on practice alongside the published academic literature and experiences drawn from our own involvement in participatory projects. While these conversations have captured the passion for social justice that drives many digital storytelling facilitators, we've also attended to our colleagues' frustrations, reflections, ironic observations, and moments of resignation about the limits and challenges of what they are trying to do. Coming to understand the work of practitioners has prompted our own learning, through listening, sharing, and collaborating across disciplinary, geographical, and cultural boundaries – as well as the boundary between work and everyday life. What, then, are the directions for further learning and research that we have identified at the end of our writing journey together here?

Directions for further research

In this book we have pulled together disparate debates, literatures, and examples of how digital storytelling is operating in health and social policy, across professional education, policymaking, service improvement, and community and place-based health. While much of the published work on listening has emerged from media studies, philosophy, or political theory, we have worked with the notion that theorising diverse listening practices in applied health and social policy settings requires interdisciplinary scholarship. In particular, we believe that we have much to learn from bringing a kaleidoscope of theory to current practice. We have begun to think through the ways that listening practices are taught, learned, and used by health educators, nurses, social and human service workers, doctors, advocates, managers, diplomats, policymakers, politicians, and planners. Our aim has been to theorise the practice arising from our case studies. There is, however, much left to do in theorising practices of using life experience narratives on a larger scale.

We are very aware of the absence of accounts of what it is like to listen to mediated life experience narratives as an "end user" in this book: that is, what it is like to be a student, trainee, policymaker, or professional who listens and responds to digital stories. We would argue for research that tracks in detail the way personal stories might be, in Iedema's (2000) terms, listened to and dynamically taken up in increasingly durable materialities of institutional policies and practices. We look forward to finding out more about the "nitty gritty" of what happens to personal stories in these settings as others build on the work we have begun here. In particular, we hope to see further explorations of how, over longer timescales, listening to personal stories in everyday contexts might shape centuries-old hierarchies of knowledge. Does attention to the meta-oratory roles of host, caretaker, and broker change the ways we analyse such encounters? Can a renewed focus on embodied, emplaced, and ecosystemic listening shed new light on the way listening unfolds in practice? We look forward to finding out more.

As co-authors, we have come to the theme of digital storytelling from different disciplinary starting points, each with her own proclivities, comfort zones, anxieties, and habits of speaking. Consequently this book aims to create a new space for talking about mediated stories: one that does not always follow the disciplinary, theoretical, or methodological contours of those who have come before us. In talking and writing about the way life stories might be listened to, we have often found tensions between our first impulses as socially, culturally, and politically embedded scholars. A key tension for us was, for example, in negotiating how to represent the ways that first-person stories are mediated and selected to be "listenable to" by decision makers. Another was how to conceptualise and represent the power of listening facilitators and brokers, relative to elite decision makers and often marginalised storytellers. We have endeavoured to embrace and name such tensions throughout the book. In our view, these differences are not random inconsistencies that could or should be ironed out. Rather, they are productive tensions that resonate within and around the very field we are trying to explore. We have mined and managed our disciplinary divergences as we have worked together, using diverse interdisciplinary tools to pry apart, theorise, and debate upon how to make sense of the diverse listening practices we have encountered. After completing this book we see that the interdisciplinary challenge of questioning and mapping listening in applied settings is perhaps one reason why other writers and practitioners have often edged away from the task. Our advice to others in this regard is: please persist!

Digital storytelling practitioners and scholars who draw on narrative methods are centrally concerned with both social justice and the irreducible and irreplaceable individual voice. Yet at the same time, the convergent theoretical frameworks that account for the movement of stories, whether dialogic understandings of knowledge production from critical traditions or post-structuralist visions of mediated and "coaxed" stories, agree that both storytelling and listening are processes of mutual imbrication and encounter. As we discussed in Chapter six, there are hidden dimensions to many of these encounters – the private quality of individual listening or the "black box" of national policymaking – that make it difficult to document their nature. In reconstructing these processes we have found ourselves revisiting the defining figures of our disciplines – the coercive institution marginalising oppressed voices or the elusive shape of a subject constituted through the words and deeds of those same institutions.

If listening is, in Susan Bickford's (1996) terms, about tolerating or even embracing dissonance, our writing process has involved difficult listening to each other's often different interpretations of these encounters. Tracing what happens in these moments has forced us to traverse the space between not only our disciplinary and theoretical groundings but also our personal experiences of practice. We hope that what has emerged from the dialogue between us as co-authors is a richer and more complex account of listening, reflecting the powerful, sometimes contradictory political undercurrents that make the idea of telling personal stories to prompt social change such a compelling project in the first place. However tricky they might be, these kinds of interdisciplinary conversations and partnerships, in which concepts, assumptions, and implications are excavated and explored with new eyes, offer promise for understanding, in all their richness and complexity, the multivalent uses of personal storytelling.

All around us, we are witnessing an explosion of ways of writing about, talking about, and capturing images of one's own life, in ever-proliferating mediated public spaces. As we write, in the middle of 2016, we see the contradictory qualities of these personal stories and their uses playing out around us. On the one hand, Twitter this week has seen an outpouring of family photographs and loving testimonies in 140 characters to attentive, wise, and beloved fathers under the hashtag #indigenousdads. These beautiful micronarratives were used to speak back to a racist cartoon published in the News Corporation broadsheet *The Australian*, which implied that sky-high levels of Indigenous incarceration, youth suicide, and abuse of children in white-dominated institutions could be laid at the door of irresponsible Indigenous fathers. On the other hand, the five-yearly Census, which could be completed online for the first time, has been mired in controversies around privacy after the Australian Bureau of Statistics decided that names and addresses would have an ongoing link to demographic detail. Online satirical news website *The Shovel* noted the irony of people sharing their concerns about the security and possible commodification of personal data via Facebook, with the headline "'Census Is Invasion of My Privacy', Man Writes on Website That Knows His Underwear Size". Practices of soliciting, telling, sharing, and listening to stories in digital spaces appear in all their variety here: as moving, resistant, coercive, commodified, bureaucratic, risky, and everyday.

It is unlikely that this flow of stories and selfies will be interrupted, or that governments, corporations, and academics will refrain from tapping it. The stories people tell online about themselves, their lives, and their health are already being "harvested" for research as well as for profit (see for example, Greaves, Ramirez-Cano, Millett, Darzi, & Donaldson, 2013). It's pressingly important, then, to develop a nuanced and multidimensional account of what it might mean to use these moving personal stories, an account that leaves behind simple dystopian fears or utopian promises, for the messy and often hard-to-fathom reality of listening to stories of other people's lives.

References

Bickford, S. (1996). *The Dissonance of Democracy*. Ithaca, NY: Cornell University Press.

Fejo-King, C., & Briskman, L. (2009). Reversing colonial practices with Indigenous peoples. In J. Allan, L. Briskman, & B. Pease (Eds.), *Critical Social Work* (pp. 105–116). Crows Nest: Allen & Unwin.

Fook, J. (2012). *Social Work: A Critical Approach to Practice*. Los Angeles, CA: Sage.

Greaves, F., Ramirez-Cano, D., Millett, C., Darzi, A., & Donaldson, L. (2013). Harnessing the cloud of patient experience: Using social media to detect poor quality healthcare. *BMJ Quality & Safety, 22*(3), 251–255. doi: 10.1136/bmjqs-2012-001527

Iedema, R. (2000). Bureaucratic planning and resemiotisation. In E. Ventola (Ed.), *Discourse and Community. Doing Functional Linguistics* (pp. 47–70). Tubingen: Narr Verlag.

Matthews, N., & Sunderland, N. (2013). Digital life-story narratives as data for policy makers and practitioners: Thinking through methodologies for large-scale multimedia qualitative datasets. *Journal of Broadcasting & Electronic Media, 57*(1), 97–114.

Index

Bold page numbers indicate figures, *italic* numbers indicate tables.

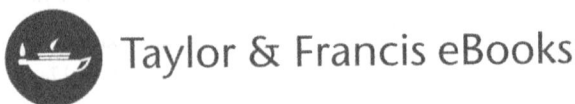
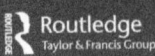